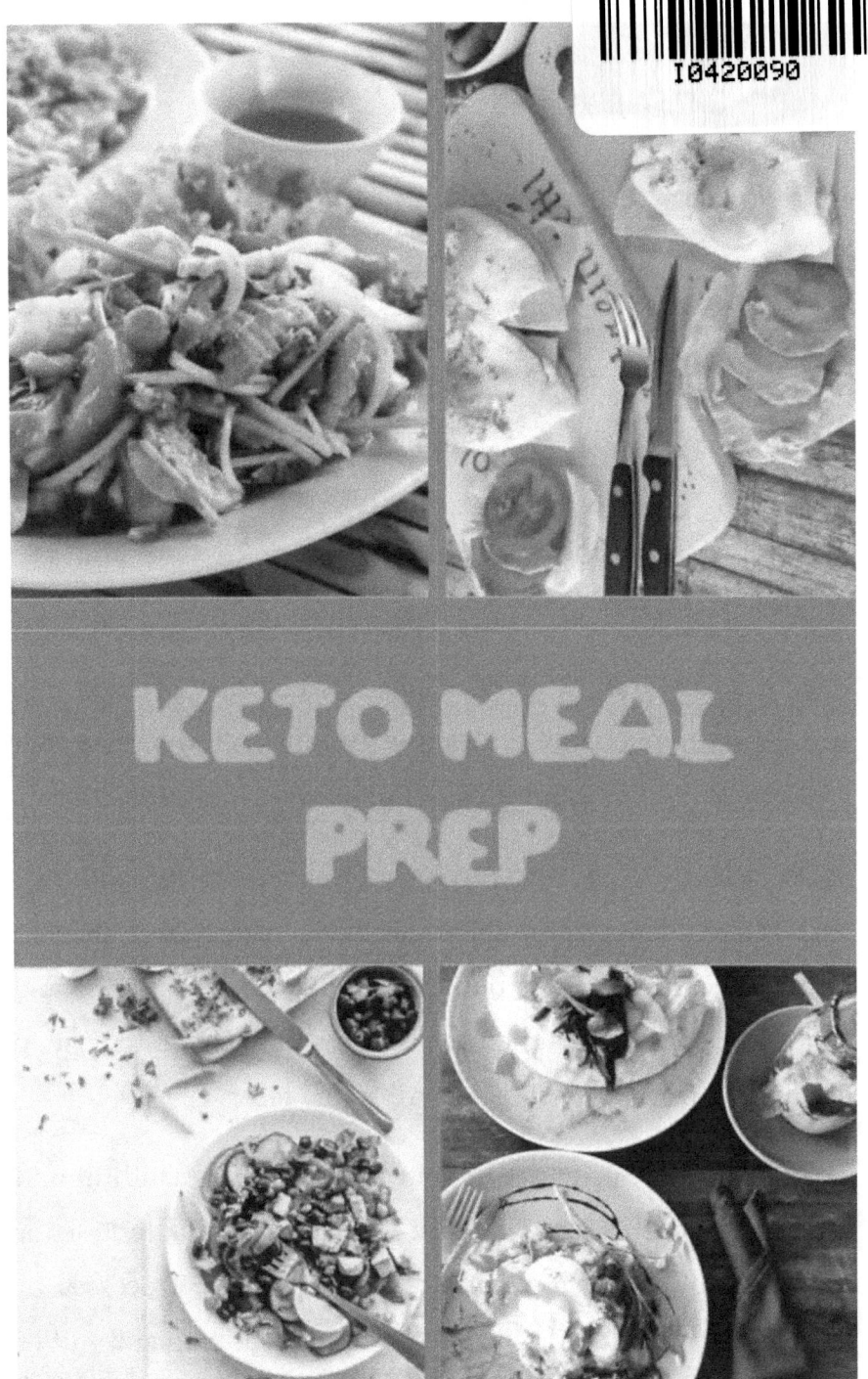

# KETO MEAL PREP

# Table Of Contents

# INTRODUCTION

The keto diet. What is the keto diet? In simple terms, it's when you trick your body into using your own BODYFAT as it's main energy source instead of carbohydrates. The keto diet is a very popular method of losing fat quickly and efficiently.

## *The Science Behind It*

To get your body into a ketogenic state you must eat a high-fat diet and low protein with NO carbs or hardly any. The ratio should be around 80% fat and 20% protein. This will the guideline for the first 2 days. Once in a ketogenic state, you will have to increase protein intake and lower fat, the ratio will be around 65% fat, 30% protein, and 5% carbs. Protein is increased to spare muscle tissue. When your body intakes carbohydrates it causes an insulin spike which means the pancreas releases insulin (helps store glycogen, amino acids and excess calories as fat) so common sense tells us that if we eliminate carbs then the insulin will not store excess calories as fat. Perfect.

Now your body has no carbs as an energy source your body must find a new source. Fat. This works out perfectly if you want to lose body fat. The body will break down the body fat and use it as energy instead of carbs. This state is called ketosis.

This is the state you want your body to be in, makes perfect sense if you want to lose body fat while maintaining muscle.

Now to the diet part and how to plan it. You will need to intake AT LEAST a gram of protein per pounds of LEAN MASS. This will help in the recovery and repair of muscle tissue after workouts and such. Remember the ratio? 65% fat and 30% protein. Well if you weight 150 pounds of lean mass which means 150g of protein a day. X4 (amount of calories per gram of protein) that is 600 calories. The rest of your calories should come from fat. If your caloric maintenance is 3000 you must eat around 500 less which would mean that if you need 2500 calories a day, around 1900 calories must come from fats! You must eat fats to fuel your body which in return will also burn off body fat! That is the rule of this diet, you must eat fats! The advantage of eating dietary fats and the keto diet is that you will not feel hungry. Fat digestion is slow which works to your advantage and helps you feel 'full'.

You will be doing this Monday - Friday and then "carb-up" on the weekend. After your last workout on Friday, this is when the carb upstarts. You must intake a liquid carbohydrate along with your whey shake post workout. This helps create an insulin spike and helps get the nutrients your body desperately needs for muscle repair and growth and refill glycogen stores. During this stage (carb up) eat what you want - pizzas, pasta, crisps, ice cream. Anything. This will be beneficial for you because it will refuel your body for the upcoming week as well as restoring your body's nutrient needs. Once Sunday starts its back to the no carb high fat moderate protein diet. Keeping your body in ketosis and burning fat as energy is the perfect solution.

Another advantage to ketosis is once you get into the state of ketosis and burn off the fat your body will be depleted of carbs. Once you load up with carbs you will look as full as ever (with less body fat!) which is perfect for the occasions on weekends when you go to the beach or parties!

## _Now lets recap on the diet._

- Must enter the state of ketosis by eliminating carbs from the diet while intaking high fat moderate/low protein.

- Must intake fibre of some sort to keep your pipes as clear as ever.

- Once in ketosis protein intake must be at least that of a gram of protein per pound of lean mass.

- That is pretty much it! It takes dedication not to eat carbs throughout the week as a lot of foods have carbs, but remember you will be rewarded greatly for your dedication.

In this eBook, you will find everything you need to know about starting the ketogenic diet, everything you need to know including the benefits and risks, plus what to eat and avoid while following a keto diet and a two-week keto meal plan to get you started.

# KETOGENIC DIETS UNDERSTANDING KETOSLS AND KETONES

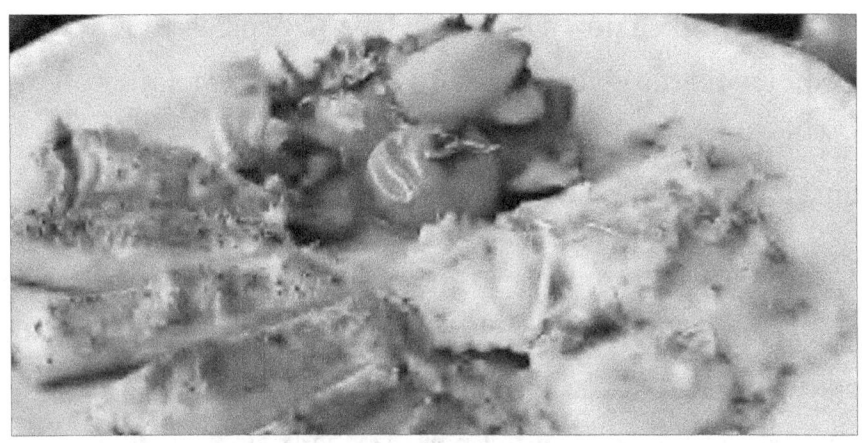

The ketogenic diet, colloquially called the keto diet, is a popular diet containing high amounts of fats, adequate protein, and low carbohydrate. It is also referred to as a Low Carb-High Fat (LCHF) diet and a low carbohydrate diet.

Ketogenic diets are basically designed to induce a state of ketosis in the body. When the amount of glucose in the body becomes too low, the body switches to fat as an alternative source of energy.

**The body has two primary fuel sources which are:**

- glucose

- free fatty acids (FFA) and, to a lesser extent, ketones made from FFA

Fat deposits are stored in the form of triglycerides. They are normally broken down into longchain fatty acids and glycerol. Stripping off the glycerol from the triglyceride molecule allows for the release of the three free fatty acid (FFA) molecules into the bloodstream to be used as energy.

The glycerol molecule goes into the liver where three molecules of it combine to form one glucose molecule. Therefore, as your body burns fat, it also produces glucose as a by-product. This glucose can be used to fuel parts of the brain as well as other parts of the body that cannot run on FFA.

However, while glucose can travel through the bloodstream on its own, cholesterol and triglycerides need a carrier to move around in the bloodstream. Cholesterol and triglycerides are packaged in a carrier called low-density lipoprotein, or LDL. Thus, the larger the LDL particle, the more triglycerides it contains.

The overall process of burning fat deposits for energy produces carbon dioxide, water, and compounds called ketones.

Ketones are produced by the liver from free fatty acids. There are composed of 2 groups of atoms linked together by a carbonyl functional group.

The body has no capability to store ketones and therefore they must be either used or excreted.

The body excretes them either through the breath as acetone or through the urine as acetoacetate.

Ketones can be used by body cells as a source of energy. Also, the brain can make use of ketones in generating about 70-75% of its energy requirement.

Like alcohol, ketones take priority as a fuel source over carbohydrates.

This implies that when they are high in the bloodstream, they must be burned first before glucose can be used as a fuel.

## What Causes Ketosis

When you start eating fewer amounts of carbohydrates, your body gets a smaller supply of glucose to use as energy compared to before.

The decrease in the number of consumed carbohydrates and the subsequent reduction in the amount of available glucose slowly forces the body to move into the state of ketosis. Thus, the body goes into a state of ketosis when there is not enough amount of glucose available to the body cells.

## Starvation Induced Ketosis

Fasting and starvation states usually involve reduced or no intake of food that the body can digest and convert into glucose. While starvation is involuntary, fasting is a more conscious choice you make to intentionally not eat.

However, the body enters into a "starvation mode" whenever you are sleeping, when you skip a meal or when you intentionally go on a fast. The lack of food intake results in a reduction in blood glucose levels. As a result, the body starts to break down its glycogen (stored glucose) stores for energy.

The glycogen is converted back into glucose and used as energy by the body.

In this state, the body also starts to burn its stored fats. Thus, the production of ketone bodies (ketogenesis) is induced by a lack of available glucose.

Any time the number of ketones in the blood outnumbers the molecules of glucose, the body cells will start making use of the ketones as their source of energy.

# MAKING KETOGENIC DIETS WORK

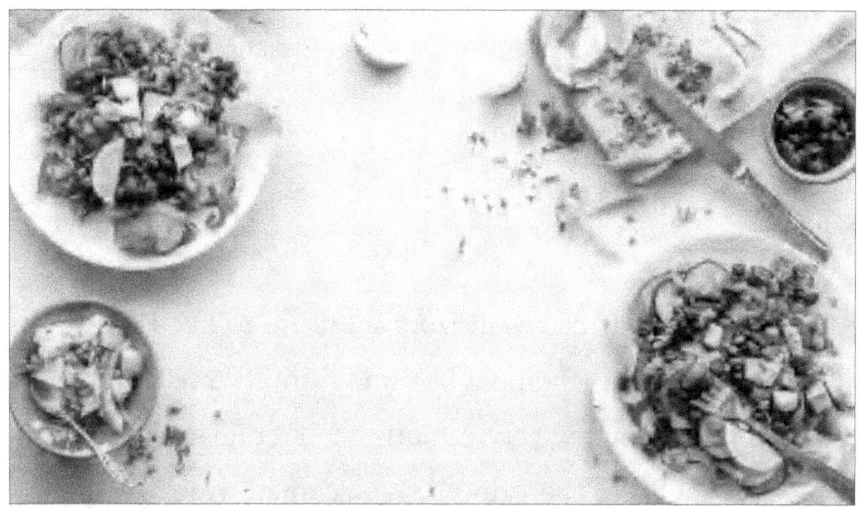

Ketogenic Diets (more specifically Cyclic Ketogenic Diets) are the most effective diets for achieving rapid, ultra low bodyfat levels with maximum muscle retention! Now, as with all such general statements, there are circumstantial exceptions. But done right - which they rarely are - the fat loss achievable on a ketogenic diet is nothing short of staggering! And, despite what people might tell you, you will also enjoy incredible high energy and overall sense of well being.

## The Perception

**Despite these promises, more bodybuilders/shapers have had negative experiences than have seen positive results. The main criticisms are:**

- Chronic lethargy

- Unbearable hunger

- Massive decrease in gym performance

- Severe muscle loss

All of these criticisms result from a failure to heed the caveat above: Ketogenic Diets must be done right! It must be realized that they are an entirely unique metabolic modality that adheres to none of the previously accepted 'rules' of dieting. And there is no going half-way; 50 grams of carbs per day plus high protein intake is NOT ketogenic!

So how are ketogenic diets 'done right'? Lets quickly look at how they work.

## Overview of Ketosis

Simply, our body, organs, muscles, and brain can use either glucose or ketones for fuel. It is the function of the liver and pancreas (primarily) to regulate that fuel supply and they show a strong bias toward sticking with glucose. Glucose is the 'preferred' fuel because it is derived in abundance from the diet and readily available readily from liver and muscle stores. Ketones have to be deliberately synthesized by the liver, but the liver can easily synthesize glucose (a process known as 'gluconeogenesis' that uses amino acids (protein) or other metabolic intermediaries) too.

We don't get beta-hydroxybutyrate, acetone, or acetoacetate (ketones) from the diet. The liver synthesizes them only under duress; as a last measure in conditions of severe glucose deprivation like starvation. For the liver to be convinced that ketones are the order of the day, several conditions must be met:

- Blood glucose must fall below 50mg/dl

- Low blood glucose must result in low Insulin and elevated Glucagon

- Liver glycogen must be low or 'empty'

- A plentiful supply of gluconeogenic substrates must NOT be available

At this point it is important to mention that it is not actually a question of being 'in' or 'out' of ketosis; we don't either totally run on ketones, or not. It is a gradual and careful transition so that the brain is constantly and evenly fuelled... ideally. Ketones SHOULD be produced in small amounts from blood glucose levels of about 60mg/dl. We consider ourselves in ketosis when there are greater concentrations of ketones than glucose in the blood.

The reality is that most people - especially weight trainers - have had a regular intake of glucose for a good couple of decades, at least. The liver is perfectly capable of producing ketones but the highly efficient gluconeogenic pathways are able to maintain low-normal blood glucose above the ketogenic threshold.

Couple this with the fact that many people are at least partially insulin resistant and have elevated fasting insulin (upper end of the normal range, anyway). The small amount of blood glucose from gluconeogenesis induces sufficient insulin release to blunt glucagon output and the production of ketones.

Sudden glucose deprivation will have the consequence, initially, of lethargy, hunger, weakness, etc in most people - until ketosis is achieved. And Ketosis will not be reached until the liver is forced to quit with gluconeogenesis and start producing ketones. As long as dietary protein is sufficient then the liver will continue to produce glucose and not ketones. That's why no carb, high protein diets are NOT ketogenic.

## What's So Great About Ketosis Anyway?

When the body switches over to running primarily on ketones a number of very cool things happen:

- Lipolysis (bodyfat breakdown) is substantially increased

- Muscle catabolism (muscle loss) is substantially reduced

- Energy levels are maintained in a high and stable state

- Subcutaneous fluid (aka 'water retention') is eliminated

Basically, when we are in ketosis our body is using fat (ketones) to fuel everything. As such, we aren't breaking down muscle to provide glucose. That is, muscle is being spared because it has nothing to offer; fat is all the body needs (well, to a large extent). For the dieter, this means substantially less muscle loss than what is achievable on any other diet. Make sense?

As a bonus, ketones yield only 7 calories per gram. This is higher than the equal mass of glucose but substantially less (22%, in fact) than the 9 calorie gram of fat from whence it came. We like metabolic inefficiencies like this. They mean we can eat more but the body doesn't get the calories.

Even cooler is that ketones cannot be turned back into fatty acids; the body excretes any excess in the urine! Speaking of which, there will be quite a bit of urine; the drop in muscle glycogen, low Insulin, and low aldosterone all equate to massive excretion of intra and extracellular fluid. For us that means hard, defined muscularity and quick, visible results.

Regarding energy, our brain actually REALLY likes ketones so we tend to feel fantastic in ketosis - clear-headed, alert and positive. And because there is never a shortage of fat to supply ketones, energy is high all the time. Usually, you even sleep less and wake feeling more refreshed when in ketosis.

Doing it Right

From whats said above you will realize that to get into ketosis:

- Carbohydrate intake should be nil; Zero!
- Protein intake should be low - 25% of calories at a maximum
- Fat must account for 75%+ of calories

With low insulin (due to zero carbs) and calories at, or below maintenance, the dietary fat cannot be deposited in adipose tissues. The low-ish protein means that gluconeogenesis will quickly prove inadequate to maintain blood glucose and, whether the body likes it or not, there is still all the damned fat to burn.

And burn it does. The high dietary fat is oxidized for cellular energy in the normal fashion but winds up generating quantities of Acetyl-CoA that exceed the capacity of the TCA cycle. The significant result is ketogenesis - synthesis of ketones from the excess Acetyl-CoA. In more lay terms: the high fat intake "forces" ketosis upon the body. This is how it's done right'.

Now you just have to throw out what you thought was true about fats. Firstly, fat does not "make you fat". Most of the information about the evils of saturated fats, in particular, is so disproportionate or plain wrong anyway; on a ketogenic diet, it is doubly inapplicable. Saturated fats make ketosis fly. And don't worry; your heart will be better than fine and your insulin sensitivity will not be reduced (there is no insulin around in the first place)!

Once in ketosis, it is not necessary, technically speaking, to maintain absolute zero carbs or low protein. But it is still better if you want to reap the greatest rewards. Besides, assuming you are training hard, you will still want to follow a cyclic ketogenic diet where you get to eat all your carbs, fruit and whatever else, every 1-2 weeks, anyway (more on this in another article).

Don't be mistaken; 'done right' does not make ketogenic dieting easy or fun for the culinary acrobats among you. They are probably the most restrictive diets you can use and not an option if you don't love animal products. Get out your nutritional almanac and work out a 20:0:80 protein:carb: fat diet. Yeah, it's boring. As an example, your writers daily ketogenic diet is 3100 Calories at 25:0.5:74.5 from only:

- 10 XXL Whole Eggs

- 160ml Pure Cream (40% fat)

- 400g Mince (15% fat)

- 60ml Flaxseed Oil

- 30g Whey Protein Isolate

## *Supplementation?*

There are a number of supplements that assist in making Ketogenic diets more effective. However, many popular supplements would be wasted. Here is an overview of the main ones:

- Chromium and ALA, while not insulin 'mimickers' as many claims, increase insulin sensitivity resulting in lower insulin levels, higher glucagon, and a faster descent into deeper ketosis

- creatine is a bit of a waste - at most, 30% can be taken up by the muscles that, without glycogen, cannot be meaningfully 'volumized'.

- HMB (if it works) would/should be an excellent supplement for minimizing the catabolic period before ketosis is achieved

16

- Tribulus is excellent and comes highly recommended as it magnifies the increased testosterone output of a ketogenic diet

- Carnitine in L or Acetyl-L form is an almost essential supplement for Ketogenic Diets. LCarnitine is necessary for the formation of Ketones in the liver.

- Glutamine, free-form essential and branched-chain aminos are worthwhile for pre and post training. Just don't overdo the glutamine as it supports gluconeogenesis

- ECA stack fat burners are very useful and important though don't worry about the inclusion of HCA

- Flaxseed oil is great but does not think that you need 50% of your calories from essential fatty acids. 1-10% of calories is more than sufficient.

- Whey Protein is optional - you don't want too much protein to remember

- A soluble fiber supplement that is non-carbohydrate based is good. But walnuts are easier.

Ketogenic diets offer a host of unique benefits that cannot be ignored if you are chasing the ultimate, low body fat figure or physique. However, they are not the most user-friendly of diets and any 'middle ground' compromise you might prefer will be just the worst of all worlds. Your choice is to do them right or not at all.

## What are macros?

The three main "macros" (macronutrients) are carbohydrates (carbs), protein, and fats.

You can use an online keto calculator to check what are the optimal macros according to your specific goals, current weight, age, gender, level of activity, etc.

- Calories from Carbs: 5-10%

- Calories from Protein: 20-25%

- Calories from Fat: 70-80%

For ideas and inspiration on how to reach your macros, take a look at our keto recipes. If you don't want to deal with the meal planning, consider getting detailed shopping lists, meal plans, and free coaching in my Keto for Accelerated Fat Loss Program.

## Different types of Keto Diets

What's the best type for you? There's no direct answer to which of these types will give you the fastest results. If you know your limits and work out intently most days of the week, then a TKD or CKD may be right for you.

The glycogen (a molecule that our bodies use as energy) stores need to be refilled on a ketogenic diet too.

Is your final goal to build muscle mass? You will need to increase your protein intake up to 1.0-1.2g. per kilo of body weight.

- **Standard Ketogenic Diet (SKD):** This is the most common diet type. It's the best approach if fat loss is your goal. The vast majority of people follow the standard ketogenic diet. Stick with less than 20g net carbs per day, moderate protein intake and up the fat intake.

- **Targeted Ketogenic Diet (TKD):** The TKD is best for people who need more energy around workouts time. An individual following the TKD approach increases the carbs before a workout.

- **Cyclical Ketogenic Diet (CKD):** The CKD means restricting carbs to a minimum for several days followed by a day or two of eating a high carb. This is called "carb-loading". This variation of the keto diet is best for bodybuilders or athletes to help with weight loss building lean mass.

## _Exercise on a Ketogenic Diet_

At the beginning of the ketogenic diet, you will notice that your energy is lower than usual. That's because you transition to a new fuel (ketones). All you need to do is to drink enough water, replenish electrolytes, and eat sufficient fat.

An exercise is a wellbeing tool before being a weight loss tool. Physical activity makes most people feel better by only getting a moderate amount of training.

**Reasons to exercise:**

- Lose weight (body fat)
- Get in shape
- Stay healthy
- Look good and feel good
- Improve strength and flexibility
- Build muscle

A 2014 study tested off-road cyclists to determine the long-term effects of the ketogenic diet on performance and exercise metabolism. They noticed favorable changes in body mass and body composition.

Numerous studies have shown that keto-adapted athletes performed better on a low carb diet and lost a significant amount of body fat.

Several recent studies have shown that CrossFit athletes can still perform well on a low carb diet while improving body composition.

One study found that after six weeks on a ketogenic diet, men and woman athletes significantly decreased body fat mass (-6.2 pounds), maintained muscle mass, and improved overall performance.

## Does eating a low carb diet cause ketoacidosis?

In fact, ketoacidosis is a life-threatening malfunction of the body, when ketone production is imbalanced and excessive. It is caused when very high blood sugar and very high levels of ketones happen simultaneously.

## Difference between ketosis and ketoacidosis

What's important to remember is that ketoacidosis is not usually seen in healthy individuals going on a ketogenic diet or even supplementing with exogenous ketones.

## What Happens To The Body

Your body is used to burn glucose for energy. When you drastically cut the carbohydrate intake, your body is confused and has to learn how to use fatty acids for energy.

When your body has to deal with the empty glucose stores, it has to create a new pack of enzymes. Adapting to the low carb lifestyle and switching from running on carbohydrates to using fat as the new fuel can take a few weeks.

Have the patience to truly keto-adapt and remember all the health benefits you will experience. Once a person is adopted, the body tends to balance out and regulate all the biological processes.

Have you ever tried a low carb diet and felt sick in the first days? A part of the transitioning to relying on fat includes some symptoms like headaches, dizziness, nausea and feeling lightheaded.

Most of the time all these symptoms suggest a lack of electrolytes, due to the diuretic effect. Along with the increased excretion of water, you also lose minerals faster. Stay hydrated and keep an eye on the sodium intake.

Salt – is the answer to beating the "keto-flu". Use sodium as much as possible as it will help with water retention and with the keeping the electrolytes at a healthy level.

### Keto Flu

Keto flu, also called 'induction flu' is the most common side effect for beginners- it makes people feel sick after 3-4 days after starting the diet. Transitioning can make you tired, dizzy, exhausted, etc.

**The main reasons for the keto flu:**

- Withdrawal from Carbs. Some studies show that sugars (carbohydrates) are as addictive as cocaine and heroin. Your body is not used to process a higher intake of fat and needs to create enzymes to be able to do this. In the withdrawal period, many people (including myself) report headaches, irritability and increased cravings for carbs. To make the transition easier, you can start by slowly reducing the carb intake. Give your body time to get used to the new fuel.

- Electrolyte imbalance. As mentioned before, keto has a diuretic effect. Every time you go to the bathroom, along with the liquids, you lots of electrolytes (sodium, magnesium, potassium). The fact is that once you reduce the carb intake, your kidneys switch from retaining salt to rapidly excreting it along with a significant amount of water. What you can do to feel better is trying to drink bouillon for extra salt, and drink my electrolyte drink during the day.

## *How long does the keto flu last?*

Drinking sufficient water (bone broth) and replenishing electrolytes, while eating more fat can realize most of the symptoms of the keto flu in less than a week. The process can take more or less depending on each person.

Bone broth also helps with maintaining a normal electrolyte level. Eating 1-2 cups of bone broth every day is essential if you want to feel energized while following a ketogenic diet.

This soup made out of bones has impressive health benefits: it reduces joint pain, helps with muscle repairs, fights colds, great for adrenal fatigue, reduces inflammation, etc.

Don't worry if you don't have enough energy to perform well in the gym as you did before starting. It is only temporary, and once you become adapted, your body will know how to use fat as the primary source of energy,

If you still find yourself in the position of not handling well the initial carb-restriction symptoms, read my keto flu guide and learn how to instantly relief them.

## *Common Side Effects on a Keto Diet*

Transitioning to a strict carb diet often comes with a few side effects that are only temporary.

Drinking enough water and including high in micronutrient foods are a great way to make the adapting to a high-fat diet easier.

Read below some of the most common side effects and know if you struggled with any of it and what cure you used to beat them.

## Muscle Cramps

Muscle cramps, usually leg cramps are pretty common in the begging of a strict ketogenic diet. It is a side effect of the diet being diuretic and increased urination. To me, it usually occurs by night time, but others get cramps in the morning. What you have to do is to drink more water, salt everything and take a magnesium supplement.

## Constipation

Being new to this diet can cause constipation, as your digestive system needs time to adapt to this lifestyle change.

Here's what you can do if you have this possible side effect.

- Drink enough water and increase the salt intake. Usually, the most common cause of constipation is dehydration. One quick and easy solution is to make sure you are drinking water and salt everything you eat.

- Increase the number of vegetables you are eating. Make sure you are getting enough vegetables to get high-quality fiber.

- Include Psyllium Seeds Husks in your diet. A trick I use and does miracles is to have one tablespoon psyllium seeds husks with a large glass of water in the evening.

## Heart palpitations keto diet

If you experience an elevated heart rate in the first few weeks of the keto diet, it's nothing to worry. Dehydration and a lack of salt can cause an elevated heart rate.

If the problem persists, you may need to add a potassium supplement to your diet.

## Reduced Physical Performance

Since your body still tries to adapt to entirely working on a completely new fuel source, you may feel weak in the first few days. Lots of studies have shown that keto diets are effective for endurance in athletes.

Just be patient, stick to eating 20-50 grams of carbs, increase the fat intake until you get your strength and energy back.

## Other Less Common Side Effects on a Keto Diet

Some people experience less common symptoms on the keto diet. Most of them are related to being hydrated and having a balanced electrolytes intake. Make sure you are getting enough water and micronutrients.

## Keto Rash

The best thing you can do, if you are affected by the keto rash is to wear clothes that absorb sweat and shower every time after physical activity.

Try increasing the carb intake enough to get you out of ketosis to see if the keto rash disappears.

## Increased Cholesterol

The classic effect of a ketogenic diet on cholesterol is a slightly increased, mostly due to an elevation of the good cholesterol (HDL), lowering risk of heart disease.

The increased triglyceride numbers are typical of people losing weight. As you get to a steady weight, the increases in the triglycerides will stop.

The cholesterol profile improves in two more ways: lower triglycerides and larger, fluffier LDL particles.

## Hair Loss

Experiencing hair loss whiting going on a new diet is a common issue, and it's only temporary.

Make sure you are not restricting your calories and eat as much fat as you need to feel good and satisfied. Eat nutrient dense, delicious foods to avoid any nutrient deficiencies.

## Indigestion

When transitioning, you may experience indigestion, stomach pain, heartburn. It might be frustrating having these issues since you are making healthier choices than before. Try to increase the fat intake slowly, make sure you are well hydrated.

## Reduced tolerance to alcohol

There is no apparent reason for this, but you'll likely tolerate less alcohol. Drinking alcohol will also slow down the weight loss process, as the body burns the alcohol before anything else.

Drinking alcohol also slows the ketone production. **How to eat cheap on keto?**

Cleaning your pantry and making space for new keto staples may seem expensive, especially in the beginning. In fact, in the long term, it's way cheaper than you may think. Few tips that help you shop smart and save money while cooking low carb meals.

- Plan your meals and make shopping lists. There's no better way to buy only the things you need than making a keto meal plan ahead. Take a look at the ingredients you already have in your kitchen, go online and find keto recipes that you will love eating the next week. Make a shopping list with all the ingredients you need, purchase them and cook.

- Buy bargains. Buying in bulk often comes with extra discounts. Finding a local butcher can also reduce costs. Buy cheaper cuts of meat, the ones higher in fat are usually less expensive than the lean meats. Meal prep your meals and use leftovers efficiently. This way you will spend less time in the kitchen and save some money.

- Eat homemade meals. Eating out can get very expensive. When cooking at home, it's easier to eat healthier, and you will most likely use higher-quality ingredients. Keep your meals super simple. Include protein, vegetables cooked in lots of healthy fats to keep you full for longer.

# USES AND BENEFITS OF
# THE KETOGENIC DIET

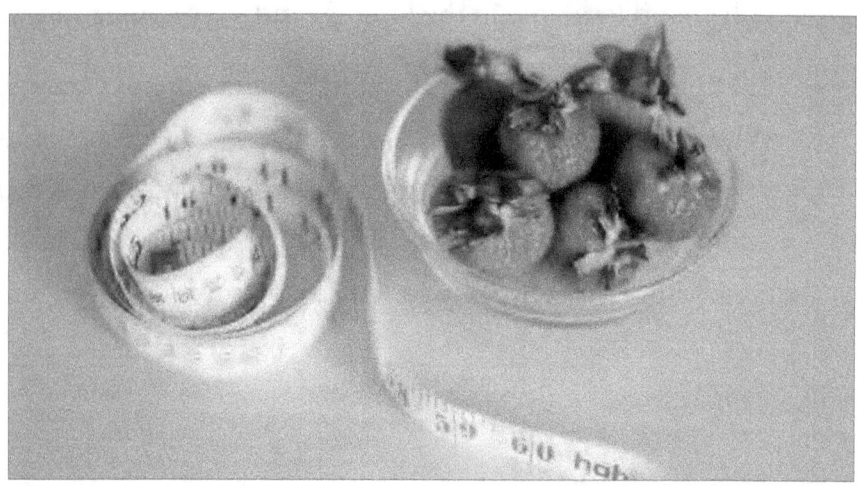

When using a ketogenic diet, your body becomes more of a fat burner than a carbohydratedependent machine. Several types of research have linked the consumption of increased amounts of carbohydrates to the development of several disorders such as diabetes and insulin resistance.

By nature, carbohydrates are easily absorbable and therefore can also be easily stored by the body. Digestion of carbohydrates starts right from the moment you put them into your mouth.

As soon as you begin chewing them, amylase (the enzymes that digest carbohydrate) in your saliva is already at work acting on the carbohydrate-containing food.

In the stomach, carbohydrates are further broken down. When they get into the small intestines, they are then absorbed into the bloodstream. On getting to the bloodstream, carbohydrates generally increase the blood sugar level.

This increase in blood sugar level stimulates the immediate release of insulin into the bloodstream. The higher the increase in blood sugar levels, the more the amount of insulin that is released.

Insulin is a hormone that causes excess sugar in the bloodstream to be removed in order to lower the blood sugar level. Insulin takes the sugar and carbohydrate that you eat and stores them either as glycogen in muscle tissues or as fat in adipose tissue for future use as energy.

However, the body can develop what is known as insulin resistance when it is continuously exposed to such high amounts of glucose in the bloodstream. This scenario can easily cause obesity as the body tends to quickly store any excess amount of glucose. Health conditions such as diabetes and cardiovascular disease can also result from this condition.

Keto diets are low in carbohydrate and high in fat and have been associated with reducing and improving several health conditions.

One of the foremost things a ketogenic diet does is to stabilize your insulin levels and also restore leptin signaling. Reduced amounts of insulin in the bloodstream allow you to feel fuller for a longer period of time and also to have fewer cravings.

## Medical Benefits of Ketogenic Diets

The application and implementation of the ketogenic diet have expanded considerably. Keto diets are often indicated as part of the treatment plan in a number of medical conditions.

## Epilepsy

This is basically the main reason for the development of the ketogenic diet. For some reason, the rate of epileptic seizures reduces when patients are placed on a keto diet.

Pediatric epileptic cases are the most responsive to the keto diet. There are children who have experience seizure elimination after a few years of using a keto diet.

Children with epilepsy are generally expected to fast for a few days before starting the ketogenic diet as part of their treatment.

## Cancer

Research suggests that the therapeutic efficacy of the ketogenic diets against tumor growth can be enhanced when combined with certain drugs and procedures under a "press-pulse" paradigm.

It is also promising to note that ketogenic diets drive the cancer cell into remission. This means that keto diets "starve cancer" to reduce the symptoms.

## Alzheimer Disease

There are several indications that the memory functions of patients with Alzheimer's disease improve after making use of a ketogenic diet.

Ketones are a great source of alternative energy for the brain especially when it has become resistant to insulin. Ketones also provide substrates (cholesterol) that help to repair damaged neurons and membranes. These all help to improve memory and cognition in Alzheimer patients.

## Diabetes

It is generally agreed that carbohydrates are the main culprit in diabetes. Therefore, by reducing the amount of ingested carbohydrate by using a ketogenic diet, there are increased chances for improved blood sugar control.

Also, combining a keto diet with other diabetes treatment plans can significantly improve their overall effectiveness.

## _Gluten Allergy_

Many individuals with a gluten allergy are undiagnosed with this condition. However, following a ketogenic diet showed improvement in related symptoms like digestive discomforts and bloating.

Most carbohydrate-rich foods are high in gluten. Thus, by using a keto diet, a lot of the gluten consumption is reduced to a minimum due to the elimination of a large variety of carbohydrates.

## _Weight Loss_

This is arguably the most common "intentional" use of the ketogenic diet today. It has found a niche for itself in the mainstream dieting trend. Keto diets have become part of many dieting regimens due to its well-acknowledged side effect of aiding weight loss.

Though initially maligned by many, the growing number of favorable weight loss results has helped the ketogenic to better embraced as a major weight loss program.

Besides the above medical benefits, ketogenic diets also provide some general health benefits which include the following.

## *Improved Insulin Sensitivity*

This is obviously the first aim of a ketogenic diet. It helps to stabilize your insulin levels thereby improving fat burning.

## *Muscle Preservation*

Since protein is oxidized, it helps to preserve lean muscle. Losing lean muscle mass causes an individual's metabolism to slow down as muscles are generally very metabolic. Using a keto diet actually helps to preserve your muscles while your body burns fat.

Controlled pH and respiratory function

A keto diet helps to decrease lactate thereby improving both pH and respiratory function. A state of ketosis, therefore, helps to keep your blood pH at a healthy level.

## *Improved Immune System*

Using a ketogenic diet helps to fight off aging antioxidants while also reducing inflammation of the gut thereby making your immune system stronger.

### Reduced Cholesterol Levels

Consuming fewer carbohydrates while you are on the keto diet will help to reduce blood cholesterol levels. This is due to the increased state of lipolysis. This leads to a reduction in LDL cholesterol levels and an increase in HDL cholesterol levels.

### Reduced Appetite and Cravings

Adopting a ketogenic diet helps you to reduce both your appetite and cravings for calorie-rich foods. As you begin eating healthy, satisfying, and beneficial high-fat foods, your hunger feelings will naturally start decreasing.

# IS THE KETO DIET RIGHT FOR YOU?

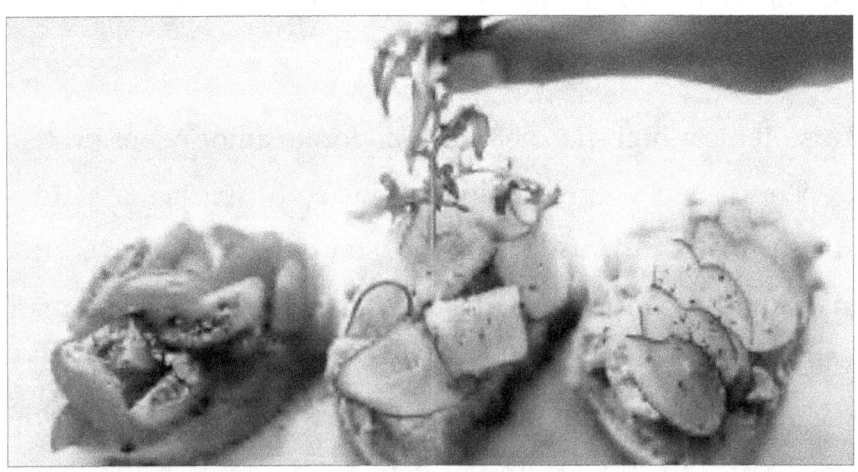

Are you interested in losing weight? Are you tired of diets that advocate low or no fats and crave your high-fat meats? You may well be considering going on the keto diet, the new kid on the block. Endorsed by many celebrities including Halle Berry, LeBron James, and Kim Kardashian among others, the keto diet has been the subject of much debate among dietitians and doctors.

**Do you wonder if the keto diet is safe and right for you?**

## *What is the ketogenic diet anyway?*

You must be aware that the body uses sugar in the form of glycogen to function. The keto diet that is extremely restricted in sugar forces your body to use fat as fuel instead of sugar, since it does not get enough sugar. When the body does not get enough sugar for fuel, the liver is forced to turn the available fat into ketones that are used by the body as fuel - hence the term ketogenic.

This diet is a high-fat diet with moderate amounts of protein. Depending on your carb intake the body reaches a state of ketosis in less than a week and stays there. As fat is used instead of sugar for fuel in the body, the weight loss is dramatic without any supposed restriction of calories. The keto diet is such that you should aim to get 60-75% of your daily calories from fat, 15-30% from protein and only 5-10% from carbohydrates. This usually means that you can eat only 2050 grams of carbs in a day.

## *What can you eat on this diet?*

The diet is a high-fat diet that is somewhat similar to Atkins. However, there is greater emphasis on fats, usually 'good' fats. On the keto diet, you can have

- Olive oil

- Coconut oil

- Nut oils

- Butter

- Ghee

- Grass-fed beef

- Chicken

- Fish

- Other Meats

- Full fat cheese □ Eggs

- Cream

- Leafy greens

- Non-starchy vegetables

- Nuts

- Seeds

You can also get a whole range of snacks that are meant for keto followers. As you can see from this list, fruits are restricted. You can have low sugar fruits in a limited quantity (mostly berries) but will have to forego your favorite fruits as these are all sweet and/or starchy.

This diet includes no grains of any kind, starchy vegetables like potatoes (and all tubers), no sugar or sweets, no bread and cakes, no beans and lentils, no pasta, no pizza and burgers, and very little alcohol. This also means no coffee with milk or tea with milk - in fact, no milk and ice-creams and milk-based desserts.

Many of these have workarounds as you can get carbohydrate free pasta and pizza, you can have cauliflower rice and now there are even restaurants that cater to keto aficionados.

## What are the benefits of the keto diet?

If you are wondering if this diet is safe, its proponents and those who have achieved their weight loss goals will certainly agree that it is safe. Among the benefits of the keto diet you can expect:

- Loss of weight

- Reduced or no sugar spikes

- Appetite control

- Seizure controlling effect

- Blood pressure normalizes in high blood pressure patients

- Reduced attacks of migraine

- Type 2 diabetes patients on this diet may be able to reduce their medications

- Some benefits to those suffering from cancer

Apart from the first four, there is not sufficient evidence to support its effectiveness or otherwise for other diseases as a lot more research is required over the long-term.

## Are there any side-effects of this diet?

When you initially start the keto diet, you can suffer from what is known as keto flu. These symptoms may not occur in all people and usually start a few days after being on the diet when your body is in a state of ketosis. Some of the side-effects are:

- Nausea
- Cramps and tummy pain
- Headache
- Vomiting
- Diarrhea and/or constipation
- Muscle cramps
- Dizziness and poor concentrations
- Insomnia
- Carbohydrate and sugar cravings

These may take up to a week to subside as your body get used to the new diet regime. You can also suffer from other problems when you start the keto diet - you may find that you have increased urination, so it is important to keep yourself well hydrated. You may also suffer from keto breath when your body reaches optimal ketosis and you can use a mouthwash or brush your teeth more frequently.

Usually, the side effects are temporary and once your body acclimatizes to the new diet, these should disappear.

## *How safe is the keto diet?*

Just like any other diet that restricts foods in specific categories, the keto diet is not without risks. As you are not supposed to eat many fruits and vegetables, beans and lentils and other foods, you can suffer from a lack of many essential nutrients. Since the diet is high in saturated fats and, if you indulge in the 'bad' fats, you can have high cholesterol levels upping your risk of heart disease.

In the long-term, the keto diet can also cause many nutritional deficiencies since you cannot eat grains, many fruits and vegetables and miss out on fiber as also important vitamins, minerals, phytonutrients and antioxidants among other things. You can suffer from gastrointestinal distress, lowered bone density (no dairy and other sources of calcium) and kidney and liver problems (the diet puts added stress on both the organs).

## Is the keto diet safe for you?

If you are willing to forego your usual dietary staples and are really keen to lose weight, you may be tempted to try out the keto diet. The biggest issue with this diet is poor patient compliance thanks to the carbohydrate restriction, so you have to be sure that you can live with your food choices. If you simply find it too difficult to follow, you can go on a version of the modified keto diet that offers more carbs.

However, the keto diet is definitely effective in helping you lose weight. According to a recent study, many of the obese patients followed were successful in losing weight. Any problems that they faced were temporary. If you do not have any significant health problems except for obesity and have been unsuccessful in losing weight following any conventional diet, the keto diet may a viable option. You must be absolutely determined to lose weight and be prepared to go on a restricted diet as specified. Even if you have any medical problems, you can take your doctor's advice and a nutritionist's guidance and go on this diet.

# IS YOUR KETO DIET CLEAN OR DIRTY?

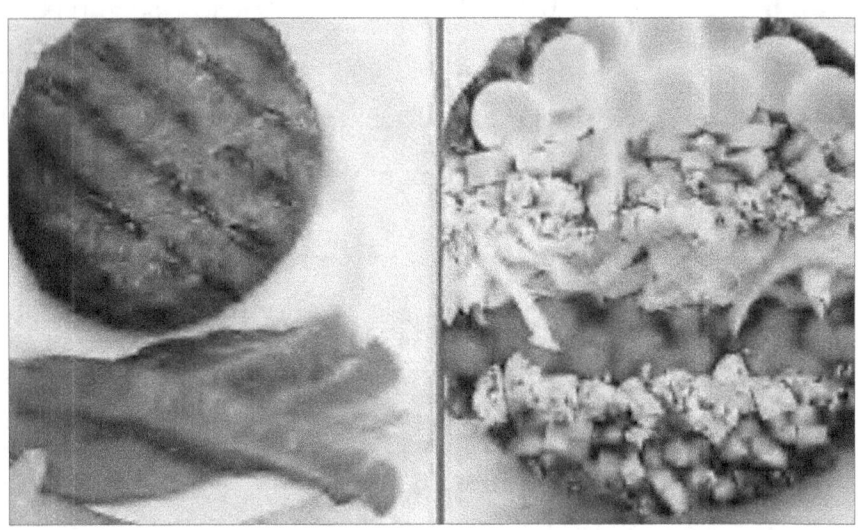

Whether you follow a keto style diet or stick to a Paleo regimen, there are good ways and bad ways to do it. A name alone does not describe a particular diet program. You can follow one to the letter, but if the foods you are using are of poor quality, you may be doing more harm than good. In this article let focus on the ketogenic (keto) diet.

A keto diet is defined as eating in a way for your body to produce ketones. Ketones are produced by the liver from fat and that process is triggered by eating very little carbohydrates and a decent amount of protein. The ketones are used by the body for energy. Thus, a keto diet essentially burns fat as the body's source of fuel. The fat is burned nonstop by your body. When your body produces ketones, it moves into a state of ketosis. The ketosis will burn fat without even worrying about fasting. That is, as long as you keep eating a ketogenic diet.

This call to mind our topic of a clean vs a dirty keto diet. Since this type of diet is limited in carbohydrates, a normal staple might be seafood, meat, and low-carb vegetables. This doesn't mean it is fine to eat a fast food burger or other commercially raised meat. If you are only just cutting your carb intake, you are living a "dirty" keto diet. The vegetables, meat, seafood, etc..., should be organic and non-GMO.

Do stay away from any processed foods or those packaged with preservatives. These will do harm to any diet and prevent you from living a toxin-free life. Any diet works best when the foods are basic and clean.

A Keto Diet has a detoxifying process when consumed properly. If you add toxins through the foods, you are not helping your liver or your health.

Eat fresh, organic vegetables. Try to regularly eat a variety of colored vegetables high in fiber. The more you do this, the better and more flavorful they will taste. Before long, your body will actually crave them for every meal.

As far as fat products, choose healthy sources. These may be organic flaxseed, olive oil, avocados, or coconut oil. Many of these are considered non-inflammatory foods. Inflammatory foods would be those such as dairy products or some of the nightshade vegetables.

While living the clean keto diet, remember to stay well hydrated. Many people do not realize that water helps all of the daily functions including digestion and organ production.

In closing, remember, if you are living the "dirty" keto diet, you're doing yourself a disservice. Stay 'clean" and stay healthy.

# KETO AND LOW-CARB RECIPE IDEAS
# 5 DELICIOUS PIZZAS FOR LOW-CARB AND KETO DIETERS

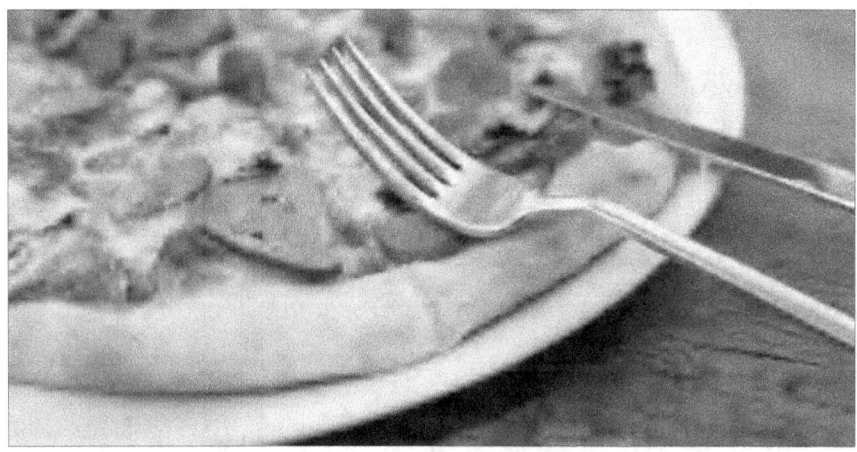

You can still eat pizza on the keto diet plan, but it takes a bit of creativity. When dining out, order a thin-crust pizza, then take your fork and slide all the toppings off the crust. It helps to order a pizza with lots of toppings. Ordering one topping on a deep dish pizza leaves you with very little left to eat.

As with most food options on keto, the best pizza is the one you make yourself. Try the low-carb pizza crust recipe, then use some of these ideas for toppings:

**Mexican pizza** - Use either traditional (low-carb) pizza sauce or enchilada sauce and top with taco-seasoned ground beef or chicken. Add a bit of salsa, chopped onions, chopped jalapeno peppers, and some hot sauce (Taco Bell hot sauce is the lowest in carbs). For some added flavor, add chopped cilantro. And top with sliced avocado after baking.

**Greek pizza** - sauce, feta cheese, red onions, olives, and how about some artichoke hearts? **Buffalo chicken pizza** – You will be thrilled to discover that Frank's red-hot buffalo wing sauce is low in carbs. If you like hot, hot, hot, use chopped grilled chicken, some onions, crumbled blue cheese, and the buffalo sauce to make a zesty pizza. Don't forget to drizzle a little blue cheese dressing over the top.

**Indian pizza** - There's a local restaurant nearby that specializes in Indian pizzas, which gave me the idea of making my own. If you choose to make this delicious option, you could use a packaged Indian food seasoning for chicken on top of the low-carb crust and add some veggies. If you want to start from scratch season some chicken with traditional Indian spices, like masala, curry powder, cumin, and any other spicy Indian seasonings you can think of. Add veggies, if desired.

**Alfredo pizza** - Use a keto diet-friendly Alfredo sauce or just spoon some out of a jar. Top with chicken or shrimp, plus garlic, parsley, Roma tomatoes - and extra parmesan cheese if you'd like.

**Of course, you can have all the traditional pizza options:**

**Meat Lovers -** Pepperoni, sausage, bacon, pork, whatever you'd like. All these are very low-carb options

**Veggie lovers** - Mushrooms, onions, tomatoes, all types of peppers, artichoke hearts... you name it, it'll taste great.

Three (or four, or five) cheese pizza - Try feta cheese, blue cheese, goat cheese, cream cheese or any other tangy cheese, in addition to -- or in place of the traditional shredded mozzarella. (Remember, many low-carb crusts are also made out of cheese. You may want to be careful about overdoing it!)

Once you have a good low-carb crust, the topping ideas are endless. Keto dieters have lots of options. The only limit is your imagination.

# TIPS FOR EXERCISING WHEN ON A KETOGENIC DIET

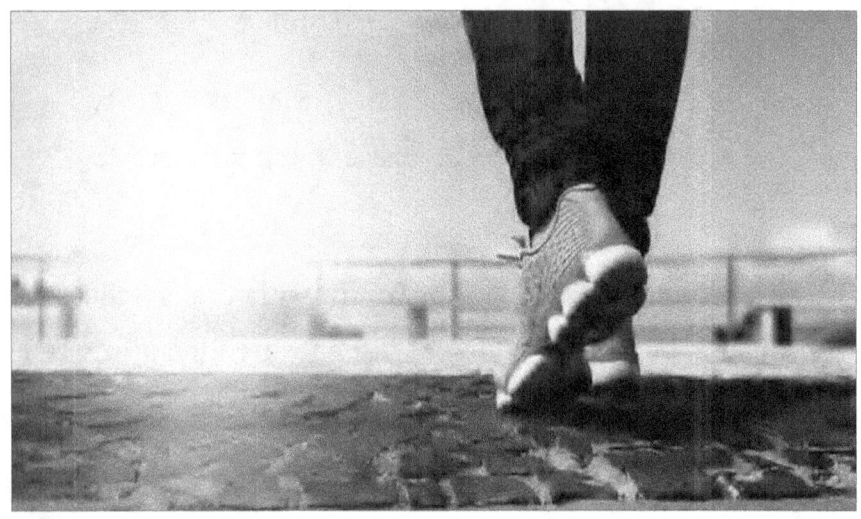

A lot of things happen when you are exercising. Some of these are good for your health and others are not so good - like when you exercise excessively.

Exercise is a stressor. While it can be a good stressor, it can, however, cause your adrenals to go into overdrive. This situation increases your insulin levels and therefore reduces your ability to lose weight.

When exercising, your insulin levels go up while your hunger reduces. However, this often results in a significant reduction in blood sugar levels which results in you becoming hungrier.

It is important to note that even a moderate increase in insulin levels causes a significant lowering of fat loss or lipolysis.

One problem we have when we want to lose weight is that we focus so much on the numbers showing on the scale. We almost unconsciously forget about the most important thing which is losing body fat.

We have more than 80 percent of our body fat stored in fat cells. To be able to get rid of this stored fat, one would need to burn it for energy production.

However, before your body can start burning your stored fats for energy, you need to be in a negative fat balance. This is a condition in which you are burning more fat off than you are actually taking in through your diet.

If your body has become used to burning fat for energy, it can now use both body fat and dietary fat for energy. This is one of the key powers of using a ketogenic diet for losing weight.

If you do not increase your dietary fat intake but increase the amount of energy your body needs through increasing your exercise intensity, your body will get almost all of that energy from burning body fat.

However, if your body is fueled with carbs, you will mostly be burning glucose for energy. This makes it a lot difficult for your body to burn and lose body fat.

It is, however, important to understand that while exercise can help you lose weight, it is more important to get the diet right first.

When you get the diet right, such a by using a well-designed ketogenic diet, your body will start tapping into its fat deposits for generating its energy. This is what effectively enables you to start burning and losing body fat.

Once your body gets used to the ketogenic diet, you will start feeling more energetic. At such a point, you will be better positioned to adjust your menus in order to start building strength and muscles.

When you get to this point during the "standard ketogenic" diet, you can then alter the diet to either a "targeted" or a "cyclical" ketogenic diet. These versions of the ketogenic diet allow more carbohydrate consumption to enable you to engage in more exercises for longer.

## Targeted Ketogenic Diet

The Targeted Ketogenic Diet allows you to ingest more carbs around your exercise period. This form of the diet allows you to engage in high-intensity exercise while still remaining in ketosis.

The carb intake within this window provides your muscles with the necessary glucose to effectively engage in your workouts. The extra glucose should normally be used up during this window of about 30 minutes and should not affect your overall metabolism.

The Targeted Ketogenic Diet is designed for beginners or intermittent exercises. The TKD allows a slight increase in your carb consumption. However, it does not kick you out ketosis and causes no shock to your system.

## Cyclical Ketogenic Diet

The Cyclical Ketogenic Diet is more appropriate for advanced athletes and bodybuilders. It is generally used for maximum muscle building results.

There is however a strong tendency for other individuals to end up adding some body fat. This is because it is easy to overeat while using the Cyclical Ketogenic Diet (CKD).

In this version of the ketogenic diet, the individual follows the standard ketogenic diet for 5 or 6 days. He or she is then allowed to eat increased amounts of carbohydrate for 1 or 2 days.

As a caution, it can take a beginner close to 3 weeks to fully get back into ketosis if he or she attempts the CKD. It requires real commitment and advanced exercise levels to successfully carry out a CKD.

The aim of the Cyclical Ketogenic Diet is to temporarily switch out of ketosis. This window gives the body the opportunity to refill the amount of glycogen in the muscles to enable it to undertake the next cycle of intense workouts.

Therefore, there must be a complete depletion of the resultant glycogen build up during the subsequent workouts in order to get back into ketosis. The intensity of your planned workout will consequently determine the amount of increased carbohydrate intake.

## *Cardio Exercises*

When you exercise at an intense rate, a lot of amazing things happen to your body.

When you engage in cardiovascular exercises, they help to improve the efficiency of your heart and lungs. This also helps to increase the rate at which your body burns energy and over time this will lead to weight loss.

Engaging in cardio exercise causes many metabolic changes that positively affect fat metabolism.

Cardiovascular exercises help to increase oxygen delivery through improved blood flow. This way, body cells are able to more effectively oxidize and burn fat.

This also has the effect of increasing the number of oxidative enzymes. Consequently, the speed at which fatty acids are transported to the mitochondria to be burned for energy is greatly increased.

During cardio exercises, the sensitivity of muscles and fat cells to epinephrine is greatly increased. This increases the number of triglycerides that are released into the blood and muscles to be burned for energy.

## *Strength Training*

Strength training helps to improve your moods while also helping to build healthy bones. It also helps you to develop an overall strong and healthy body.

Using a well-designed ketogenic will help you preserve your muscles even when carrying our strength training. Muscles are built with protein and not fat or carbs. Also, given the fact that protein oxidation is less in a ketogenic diet, engaging in strength training should not be a problem.

You need to challenge your body with heavy weights to really see results and get a stronger body.

## *Interval Training*

Interval training is simply alternating intervals of high-intensity and low-intensity workouts. It is simply for you to: go fast, go slow, and repeat.

While sounding so simple, interval training is one of the most powerful ways to burn body fat quickly. Apart from burning fat while carrying out interval training, the "afterburn effect" stimulates your metabolism for a longer period of time.

## *Circuit Training: Cardio + Strength*

Circuit training is basically the combining of cardiovascular exercises with strength training exercises. This combination helps to provide all-over fitness benefits.

This form of exercising combines cardio exercises such as jogging and a resistance workout without allowing a resting period between them. The lack of rest in-between both exercises make circuit training as effective as a cardio-based high-intensity interval training workout.

## Yoga

The exercise benefits of yoga really come from its ability to help the body reduce levels of stress hormones and also increase insulin sensitivity.

Yoga helps you to consciously connect with your body. This connection can translate into you being more mindful of how your body works and changing even your eating habits.

# ALPHA KETO-GLUTARATE

The Krebs Cycle is a chemical reaction in the body that converts fats, carbohydrates, and proteins to carbon dioxide and water which in turn gets transformed into usable energy. Although not well knows the physiological process to laymen, it is one of the most important cellular function of the body. This chemical process takes place in every cell. When severe inflammation occurs, the mitochondria, which are the actual power producing part of the cells, have an excess of nitric acid which restricts their ability to produce energy. Alpha Keto-Glutarate (AKG) is able to bypass this and enhance mitochondrial energy production thus providing increased levels of energy. But AKG does much more than this. The benefits of AKG to the human body are varied and to understand what exactly the benefits of increasing AKG levels in the body are, read on.

- When glucose or sugar molecules become attached to a protein it becomes one of the causes of diabetic vision impairment and the formation of cataracts. AKG helps to prevent this process.

- During times of strenuous exercise, the body produces plasma lactates and buffering ammonia which drain energy. AKG decreases their production and is thus an ideal supplement for an athlete who requires a short intense burst of energy, such as for short or medium distance sprints and jumps.

- Poor mitochondrial function is a major reason for chronic tiredness. Chronic tiredness is not just a lack of energy, it is a sickness. People with this problem benefit greatly from the additional intake of AKG since it both directly enhances energy production and also increases the energy-producing powers of the mitochondria and provides more energy to the body.

- The main problem with low energy production in the body is that the Krebs Cycle requires a great deal of energy to function properly. But if the body lacks energy, the Krebs Cycle cannot function properly. A real chicken and egg situation. Since AKG bypasses the blocks in the Krebs Cycle, it allows for a higher level of energy production which is partly used by the Krebs Cycle itself to function better and itself produce more AKG. AKG has the additional benefit of increasing the oxygen uptake of the mitochondria which in turn allows them to function even more efficiently.

- AKG is of benefits to diabetics who are on insulin therapy. Since it enhances the effects of insulin, the diabetics can lower their intake. In fact, they must do so; failing which they may suffer from hypoglycemia or low blood sugar complications. Another benefit of AKG for diabetics and people with high blood sugar levels or those on medically advised refined carbohydrate diets is that it inhibits protein binding. Protein binding happens when high blood sugar levels cause the sugars to bind with essential proteins that the body needs and causes them to become inactive. This increases the chances of getting diseases and also speeds up the aging process.

- Because AKG increases the heart's ability to produce the energy it is an important nutrient in the case of any problems or sicknesses that put greater pressure on the heart.

- AKG also promotes the performance of the heart when it is under stress while playing sports. Besides allowing the more efficient functioning of the heart and thus improving the bodies. Athletic performance, it also inhibits the production of lactic acid in the muscles which are the cause of the burning sensations in the muscles that are often felt after strenuous exercise.

- Besides increasing energy levels in the body, AKG also plays a role in the removal of unwanted substances from the body. Ammonia is toxic and must not be allowed to remain in the body tissue. Ammonia levels in the body increase when there is chronic fatigue or at times of high physical stress and inhibits the natural production of AKG. AKG binds with ammonia and detoxifies the tissues. But when the Ammonia itself causes a lower production of AKG by the mitochondria, we return to the chicken and egg situation. The solution lies in ingestion of AKG supplements which will detoxify the Ammonia and at the same time provide an increase in the AKG levels that are needed for the Krebs Cycle so the body produces more AKG. If you feel that this is a confusing never ending circle, the way to break it is to consume more AKG.

- AKG Also improves liver function by reducing the accumulation of toxic acids and Ammonia in the organ.

- And if all this wasn't enough, AKG is also proven to fight against cataract formation in the eyes and also help to overcome the problem of being unable to move the eye.

- And there is yet more. AKG possesses many antioxidant properties that make it a good general purpose supplement to promote overall good health.

A study done by the University of Queensland on the effects of AKG on athletes was done by giving a group of trained cyclists 4 liters of water in which certain amino acids were mixed and making them cycle till the point of exhaustion. The test was repeated a second time, but in this instance, AKG was added to the water instead of the amino acids. The result was that the second test showed a 6 to 8% improvement in the performance of the cyclists which, in sporting terms, is massive.

To start taking AKG to begin with one capsule of 1 gm every day and slowly work it up, over a period of a couple of weeks, to 2 capsules three times a day. The capsules should be taken at the beginning of each meal. Underdosing is a false economy that will result in not getting the expected results. Once these results are achieved, it should be possible to reduce the dosage to 1 capsule two or three times a day.

AKG supplements are safe and side effects are rare. However, if you do feel any form of discomfort while taking the AKG, consult a medical practitioner.

# THE BENEFITS OF MIXING MCT OIL INTO YOUR KETOGENIC DIET PLAN

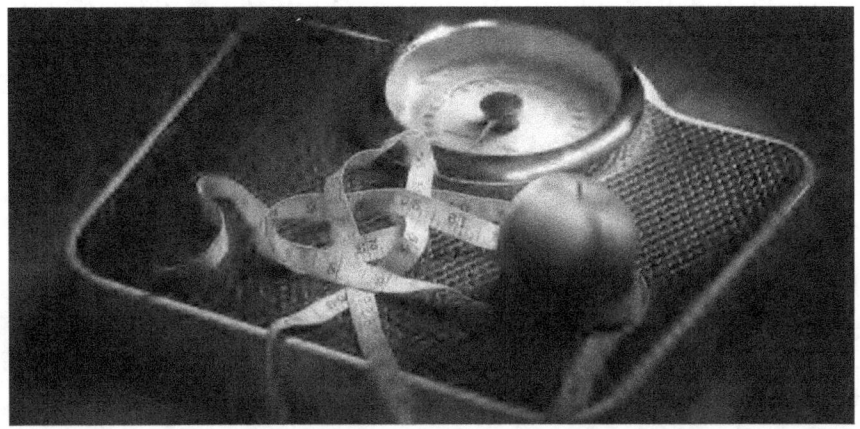

In life, we're always talking about must-haves. If you're driving a high-end car, you must have the top of the line motor oil coursing through its cylinders. If you're competing at a high level in a track competition, state of the art running shoes is a must-have. When you're celebrating a huge quarter at the office, the finest bourbon is a must have. If you're serious about a ketogenic lifestyle, MCT Oil is a must-have.

MCT Oil provides a heavy dose of the very fuels that turn your body into - and keep it - a fat burning machine. Unlike LCTs, MCTs bypass much of the digestion process that others fats go through. MCTs act in an almost carb-like manner in how they're sent directly to the liver, where they are used for energy.

There are many reasons why MCT makes perfect sense for your Ketogenic Diet, but help you understand how they can play an essential role in your nutrition, we've some of the main benefits of MCT Oil in your Ketogenic Diet plan.

## _Mct Oil Helps You Get Into Ketosis Faster_

As you already know, MCTs go to your liver and act in a "carb-like" manner that LCTs do not have the ability to do. This means that you can theoretically kickstart Ketosis by following these steps:

## _1. Fast with no breakFAST._

If you've been out of Ketosis for awhile and you want to efficiently get back into a fat burning state, a mix of fasting and MCT Oil will do the job. Just eat a very low carb dinner, or even skip dinner, and then wake up and don't eat breakfast! Instead, drink a cup of coffee, and put a tablespoon or two of MCT Oil into your coffee and head out!

The shot of MCT, plus the already fasted state of your body will have you back into Ketosis quicker than if you tried to just slowly eat your way back into Ketosis (i.e. nutritional Ketosis). It's also worth adding that the energy you get from the MCT

Oil and the coffee will be unlike what you were used to the MCTs provide prolonged energy that isn't comparable to energy derived from glycogen.

## 2. Meal replacement with MCT Oil

Another benefit that comes from using MCT Oil in your Ketogenic Diet plan is using it as a meal replacement.

This somewhat resembles the previous point of fasting with MCT Oil, but the difference is that you're still eating other regular Ketogenic meals, except your replacing (at least) one of those meals with some MCT Oil.

One of the benefits of MCT Oil is its ability to satiate your appetite. So while it sounds initially scary to just depend on a few tablespoons of oil for a meal replacement, your body will become accustomed as you do it more and more. The MCTs will act as a replacement for what's normally there (glycogen) and your fierce-badger-hunger cravings will lessen.

In our fast-paced, 21st century lifestyle, the benefits of being able to remain in Ketosis while only slurping a few tablespoons of MCTs cannot be overstated.

## 3. Ramp up your Ketogenic dishes with MCT

MCT Oil's versatility is amazing. Let's say you're already in Ketosis, but you're about to eat a salad for your daily carbs, and you want to keep it 100 on the Keto life. It's easy! Just use MCT for a base to your dressing, and you can rest assured that you'll still be burning fat after you've downed your greens!

Another way to use MCTs in your favorite Ketogenic meals is to use it as a replacement for regular oil in baking! There's a whole ocean of Keto baking recipes out there, so why not double down and use MCT instead of regular coconut oil?!

But what if you're not baking? What if you're out for a jog and you want to implement the energy efficiency of MCT Oil? How about a nice Keto "sports drink"?! All you have to do is it to water, and then squeeze in some lemon juice, and you'll have a healthier, non-sugary sports drink for long workouts in the sun!

There are many ways to skin a cat, and there are also many ways to amplify your Ketogenic Diet. MCTs are essential to your body transforming into a fat burning machine. Unfortunately, you're not always going to be able to get the proper amounts from a diet alone - you'll need a boost, and MCT Oil is that boost.

Life is full of "must haves," and your diet does not fall out of the realm of this mantra. If you want to live a truly Ketogenic lifestyle, you're going to have invested in the right fuels, and implement them in the most efficient ways possible. So what's the benefit of MCT to your Ketogenic Diet plan? The answer: efficiency. An efficient diet, which feeds an efficient lifestyle, that ultimately gives you more time to do the things you love.

# TYPE 2 DIABETES - DOES A KETO DIET HELP LOWER BLOOD SUGAR LEVELS?

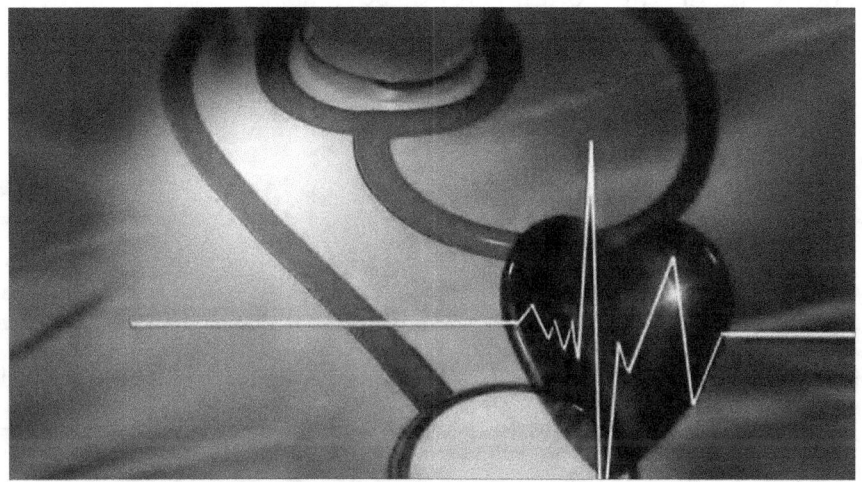

Is a ketogenic diet safe for people who have received a diagnosis of Type 2 diabetes? The food recommended for people with high blood sugar encourages weight loss: a ketogenic diet has high amounts of fat and is low in carbs, so it is mystifying how such a high-fat diet is an option for alleviating high blood sugar.

The ketogenic diet underlines a low intake of carbohydrates and increased consumption of fat and protein. The body then breaks down fat by a process called "ketosis," and produces a source of fuel called ketones. Usually, the diet improves blood sugar levels while decreasing the body's need for insulin. The diet initially was developed for epilepsy treatment, but the kinds of food and the eating pattern it highlights, are being studied for the benefit of those with Type 2 diabetes.

The ketogenic diet contains foods such as...

- pasta,
- fruits, and
- bread

As a source of body energy. People with Type 2 diabetes suffer from high and unstable blood sugar levels, and the keto diet helps them by allowing the body to preserve their blood sugar at a low healthy level.

How does a keto diet help many with Type 2 diabetes? In 2016, the Journal of Obesity and Eating Disorders published a review suggesting a keto diet may help people with diabetes by improving their A1c test results, more than a calorie diet.

The ketogenic diet places emphasis on the consumption of more protein and fat, making you feel less hungry and therefore leading to weight loss. Protein and fat take longer to digest than carbohydrates and helps to keep energy levels up.

In a nutshell, the ketogenic diet...

- lowers blood sugar,

- enhances insulin sensitivity and

- promotes less dependency on medications.

The Keto Diet Plan. Ketogenic diets are stringent, but if adhered to correctly they can provide a nourishing and healthful nutrition routine. It is about staying away from carbohydrate foods likely to spike blood sugar levels.

People with Type 2 diabetes are often advised to focus on this diet plan as it consists of a mix of low carbohydrate foods, high-fat content, and moderate protein. It is also important because it avoids high-processed foods and indulges in lightly processed and healthy foods.

A ketogenic diet should consist of these types of food...

- Low-carb vegetables: eat vegetables with every meal. Avoid starchy vegetables like corn and potatoes.

- eggs: they contain a low amount of carbohydrates and are a high source of protein.

- Meats: eat fatty meats but avoid excessive amounts. High amounts of protein plus low carbohydrates can lead to the liver converting protein into glucose, thus causing the person to come out of ketosis.

- Fish: an excellent source of protein.

Eat from healthy sources of fat like avocados, seeds, nuts, and olive oil.

It is helpful to go by what your body requires rather than what you feel you need. Always follow your doctor's advice on nutrition and medications and check with him/her before starting a new eating plan.

Although managing your disease can be very challenging, Type 2 diabetes is not a condition you must just live with. You can make simple changes to your daily routine and lower both your weight and your blood sugar levels. Hang in there, the longer you do it, the easier it gets.

# WHAT CAN YOU AT ON A KETOGENIC DIET? LEARN THE SECRETS TO BURN FAT

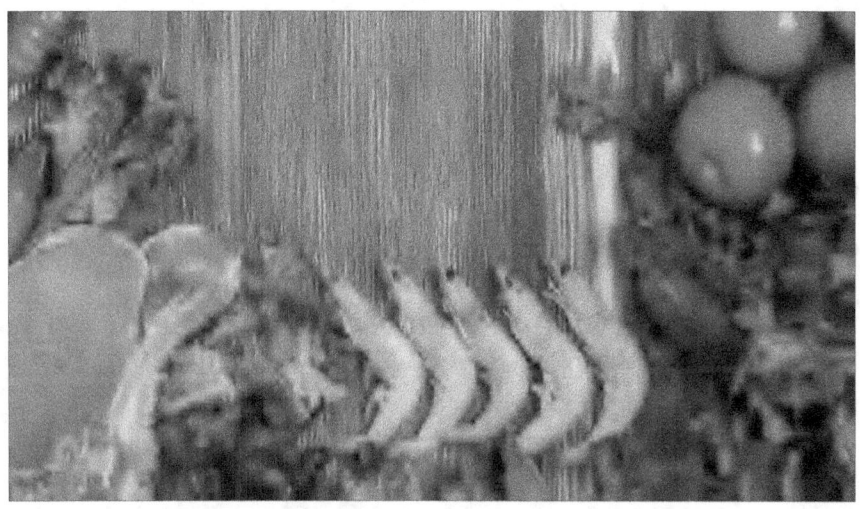

A ketogenic diet is basically a diet which converts your body from burning sugar to burning fat. Around 99% of the world's population have a diet which causes their body to burn sugar. As a result, carbohydrates are their primary fuel source used after digesting carbs. This process makes people gain weight, however, a diet of fat and ketones will cause weight loss. As you ask what can you eat on a ketogenic diet, first of all, eat up to 30 to 50 grams of carbs per day. Next, let us discover more about what you can have on your plate and how the ketogenic diet affects your health.

## The Importance Of Sugar Precaution On The Ketogenic Diet

Keto shifts your body from a sugar burner to a fat burner by eliminating the dietary sugar derived from carbohydrates. The first obvious reduction you should make from your current diet is sugar and sugary foods. Although sugar is a definite target for deletion, the ketogenic diet focuses on the limitation of carbohydrates. We need to watch out for sugar in a number of different types of foods and nutrients. Even a white potato which is carb-heavy may not taste sweet to your tongue like sugar. But once it hits your bloodstream after digestion, those carbs add the simple sugar known as glucose to your body. The truth is, our body can only store so much glucose before it dumps it elsewhere in our system. Excess glucose becomes what is known as the fat which accumulates in our stomach region, love handles, etc.

## Protein And It's Place In Keto

One source of carbohydrates which some people overlook in their diet is protein. Overconsumption of protein according to the tolerance level of your body will result in weight gain. Because our body converts excess protein into sugar, we must moderate the amount of protein we eat. Moderation of our protein intake is part of how to eat ketogenic and lose weight. First of all, identify your own tolerance of daily protein and use as a guide to maintaining an optimal intake of the nutrient. Second, choose your protein from foods such as organic cage-free eggs and grass-fed meats. Finally, create meals in variety that are delicious and maintain your interest in the diet. For instance, a 5-ounce steak and a few eggs can provide an ideal amount of daily protein for some people.

## *Caloric Intake On The Ketogenic Diet*

Calories are another important consideration for what can you eat on a ketogenic diet. Energy derived from the calories in the food we consume help our body to remain functional. Hence, we must eat enough calories in order to meet our daily nutritional requirements. Counting calories is a burden for many people who are on other diets. But as a ketogenic dieter, you don't have to worry nearly as much about calorie counting. Most people on a low-carb diet remain satisfied by eating a daily amount of 1500-1700 kcals in calories.

## *Fats, The Good & The Bad*

Fat is not bad, in fact, many good healthy fats exist in whole foods such as nuts, seeds, and olive oil. Healthy fats are an integral part of the ketogenic diet and are available as spreads, snacks, and toppings. Misconceptions in regards to eating fat are that a high amount of it is unhealthy and causes weight gain. While both statements are in a sense true, the fat which we consume is not the direct cause of the fat which appears on our body. Rather, the sugar from each nutrient we consume is what eventually becomes the fat on our body.

## *Balance Your Nutrients Wisely*

Digestion causes the sugars we eat to absorb into the bloodstream and the excess amount transfer into our fat cells. High carbohydrate and high protein eating will result in excess body fat because there is sugar content in these nutrients. So excessive eating of any nutrient is unhealthy and causes weight gain. But a healthy diet consists of a balance of protein, carbohydrates, and fats according to the tolerance levels of your body.

Just about everyone can accomplish a ketogenic diet with enough persistence and effort. In addition, we can moderate a number of bodily conditions naturally with keto. Insulin resistance, elevated blood sugar, inflammation, obesity, type-2 diabetes are some health conditions that keto can help to stabilize. Each of these unhealthy conditions will reduce and normalize for the victim who follows a healthy ketogenic diet. Low-carb, high-fat and moderate protein whole foods provide the life-changing health benefits of this diet

# FOODS YOU CAN EAT ON A KETOGENIC DIET FOR WEIGHT LOSS

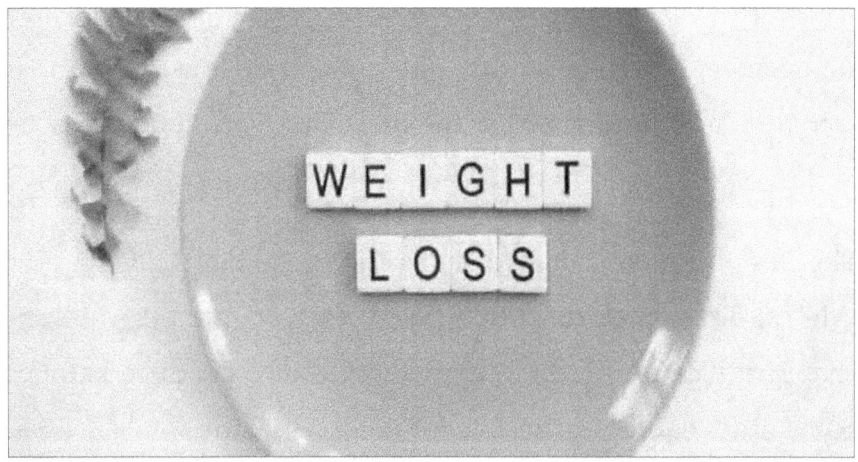

While on a ketogenic diet, it is very important to ensure that one eats within the restrictions of the diet. This is vital so as for the individual to be able to remain in a state of ketosis.

Going out of ketosis can be as simple as eating one or two meals that are not recommended on the diet. However, coming back into ketosis is another different story entirely. This can often take days or weeks depending on how strict you become when you get back on the diet.

Meals in a ketogenic diet comprised of three basic food types. These are the:

- fruit or vegetable

- protein-rich food

- fat source

## *Fats*

Ketogenic diets by nature involve the consumption of increased amounts of fats in the diet. They can come in as part of the cooking process or as sauces and dressings.

The best types of fats are those medium-chain triglycerides (MCTs). These include both MCT oil and coconut oil. Medium-chain triglycerides are easily metabolized to produce ketones. Some other equally good fats for ketosis include:

- Omega-3 and Omega-6 fatty acids

- Salmon, Shellfish, Trout, Tuna

- Monounsaturated and Saturated Fats

- Olive oil, Avocado, Butter, Cheese, Red palm oil, Egg yolks

- Non-hydrogenated oils (when cooking)

- Coconut oil, Beef tallow, Non-hydrogenated lards

- High oleic

- Safflower oils, Sunflower oils

- Other fat sources:

- Chicken skin, Coconut butter, Peanut butter, Fat on meats

- Proteins

When buying your protein foods, always try to choose grass-fed, organic and humanely raised meat and wild-caught seafood. Apart from offering more nutrients, they have not been exposed to added hormones, antibiotics, and other potential toxins.

## Meat

The ketogenic diet accepts basically any type of meat. There is no discrimination about the type of cut or preparation.

Beef, Goat, Lamb, Pork, Veal, Venison

## Poultry

Any type of poultry is also allowed by the diet. You can improve the content of the meal by leaving the skin on. However, breading and batter should not be used in the preparation of poultry as they are usually high in carbohydrates. Other than that, you can prepare your poultry to your liking.

Chicken, Duck, Game hen, Goose, Ostrich, Partridge, Pheasant, Quail, Squab, Turkey **Seafood**

Another great source of protein is seafood. Seafood is a great source of omega-3 fatty acids. They also have high amounts of minerals and vitamins to help keep you well-nourished and healthy.

Clams, Crab, Lobster, Mussels, Oysters, Prawns, Scallops, Shrimp, Snails **Fish**

Fish have good amounts of omega-3 fatty acids. You should go for fish that are caught in the wild and also in mercury-free areas.

Ahi, Catfish, Cod, Flounder, Halibut, Herring, Lobster, Mackerel, Mahi Mahi, Mussel, Salmon,

Sardines, Scallops, Snapper, Squid, Swordfish, Trout, Tuna, Walleye

## *Carbohydrates*

### Vegetables

Vegetables are the primary source of carbohydrate on a ketogenic diet. When you are buying vegetables always opt for the organically grown vegetables. Also, the dark leafy vegetables contain the least amount of carbohydrates with good nutritional value.

Arugula, Asparagus, Bok choy, Broccoli, Cabbage, Cauliflower, Celery, Collard greens, Endive, Garlic, Kale, Kelp, Lettuce, Mushrooms, Onions, Peppers, Radishes, Seaweed, Spinach, Swiss chard, Watercress

## Milk and Dairy Products

These are very essential in a ketogenic diet. The grass-fed and organic source are more preferable. The full-fat variety is better suited for the ketogenic diet than the fat-free and low-fat verities.

Butter, Cheddar, Crème fraîche, Heavy cream, Mozzarella, Sour cream, Cream cheese, Mascarpone cheese, Cheeses, Hard cheeses

## Nuts

Moderate amounts of nuts and seed are allowed on the ketogenic diet. Nuts and seed are rich in protein, fats, and carbohydrates. The total fat, protein and carbohydrate content of the nut varieties should be checked and added to the total daily calorie calculation.

Roasted nuts and seeds are the best. Anything that may cause harm or interfere with ketosis in the body has been removed from them through the roasting process.

Nuts should be used mostly as a snack

Almonds, Macadamia, and Walnuts are some of the best

Some nuts have a high content of omega-6 fatty acid which can cause inflammation in the body

However, they can hold some people back from their goals. If your weight loss is purely your purpose of using the ketogenic diet, then it would be advisable to remove nuts and seeds to improve your results.

Almonds, Brazil nuts, Hazelnuts, Pine nuts, Macadamia nuts, Pecans, Pili nuts, Pumpkin seeds, Sesame seeds, Sunflower seeds, Walnuts

## _Herbs and Spices_

After some time on the ketogenic diet, the foods may start to become boring. Adding spices to your meals can however help to spice things up. You can add fresh and dry spices to your meals and even beverages so that they become more enticing and exciting to the palate.

Spices and fresh herbs are some of the most nutrient-dense foods on the planet you can eat. Adding spices to your meal doesn't only add more flavors to the meals but also offer a lot of various health benefits to your body.

Spices contain carbohydrates thus you should ensure to add them to your daily carbohydrate count. Also, endeavor to check the labels of pre-made spice mixes for their accurate carbohydrate content as they usually contain added sugars.

Salt also enhances flavors. It is best you chose high-quality sea salt instead of traditional table salt. Unprocessed salts such as Celtic or Himalayan sea salt provide you with more than eight trace minerals that your body need to perform optimally.

Anise, Annatto, Basil, Bay leaf, Black pepper, Caraway Cardamom, Cayenne pepper, Celery seed, Chervil, Chili pepper, Chives, Cilantro, Cinnamon, Cloves, Coriander, Cumin, Curry, Dill, Fenugreek, Galangal, Garlic, Ginger, Lemongrass, Licorice, Mace, Marjoram, Mint, Mustard seeds, Oregano, Paprika, Parsley, Peppermint, Rosemary, Saffron, Sage, Spearmint, Star anise, Tarragon, Thyme, Turmeric, Vanilla beans

## Sweeteners

Adding artificial sweeteners to your meals can help in curbing cravings for carbohydrates and sweets. Sweeteners help a lot of people to be able to adhere to the ketogenic diet.

However, natural sweeteners such as honey, maple syrup, and agave raise blood sugar levels which do not only cause inflammation but can also kick you out of ketosis.

Always go for the liquid form of sweeteners as they do not have binders like dextrose and maltodextrin. Dextrose is an anti-caking agent and is a form of sugar. Maltodextrin, on the other hand, is a bulking agent which has a higher glycemic index (110) than table sugar (52).

The following is a list of recommended sweeteners which have little effect on blood sugar.

Allulose, Blended sweeteners (Swerve, Lakanto, Sukrin), Erythritol, Monk fruit, Stevia, Stevia glycerite (a thick liquid form of stevia), Sucralose, Xylitol

## Beverages

Using a low carbohydrate diet like the ketogenic diet has a diuretic effect on the body. Carbohydrates draw water to them which cause water retention in the body. However, the reduced carbohydrate intake in a ketogenic diet leads to a lot of water loss as less water is retained in the body and more is excreted.

This diuretic effect can easily lead to dehydration. Therefore you need to drink a lot of water - well above the recommended intake of 8 glasses - when you are on a ketogenic diet. This will help you to reduce the risk of bladder pain and urinary tract infections.

Besides water, you can add other types of beverages like coffee and teas to help keep you hydrated throughout the day. Both of these do not significantly affect the ketosis state.

However, the added substances like sugar and milk might affect the ketosis state. As a result, it would be best to avoid the sugar completely and use either full cream or artificial sweeteners together with your coffee or tea.

Another way to increase your beverage intake is to make vegetable juice by combining varieties of the approved vegetable types. You can also use power smoothies or protein shakes instead of fruit smoothies as the fruits contain sugars (fructose) that can kick you out of ketosis.

Below are some additional beverages you can consume to help keep you hydrated:

Unsweetened almond milk, Unsweetened cashew milk, Unsweetened coconut milk, Unsweetened hemp milk, Green tea, Herbal tea, Organic caffè Americano (espresso with water), Mineral water

# LOW CARB FOOD YOU CAN INCLUDE IN YOUR DIET

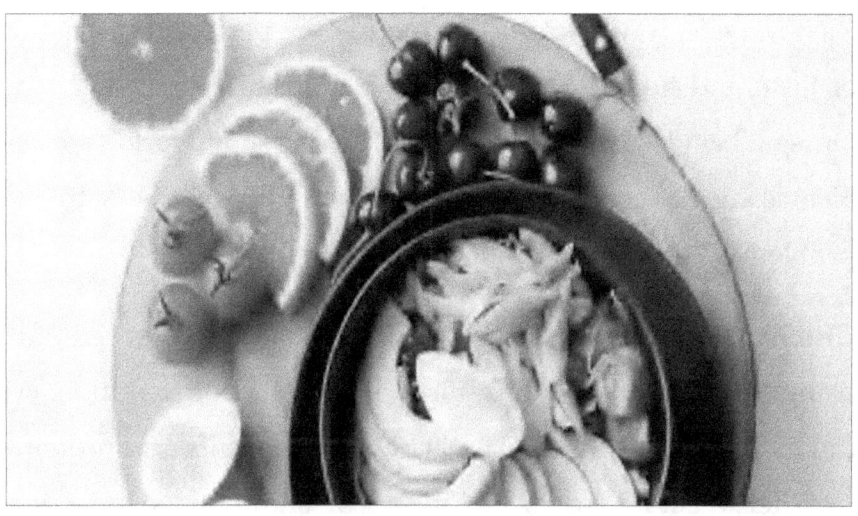

Thanks to all the fitness and yoga campaigns, health has become a priority for people as it should have been long ago. Many people are taking small but sure steps towards the fitness zone, and many are already on the road to a healthy heart. Food plays an important role in maintaining your health. People now prefer food with low carbs and fat to escape the few extra Kgs. Let's take a look at what you can eat if you want both taste and health. All these foods are low in carbs and you will not put on weight by eating these.

**Onions -** You must be surprised to see this name on the list, but you must know that onions have only 9% carbs in them. Apart from it, onions are also high in fiber. Onion work in many ways, as an antioxidant, improves flavor and has various anti-inflammatory compounds. Try to add in most meals. Seafood - Rich in taste, low in carbs, Seafood is the perfect combination of taste and health. Seafood is also high in Iodine, B-12, and Omega 3 acids. The nutritional value of fish is world famous. Fish is also recommended by doctors for people with eye problems. You can also consume them grilled.

**Chicken -** You can add chicken to your diet, rest assured of its being low in carbs. Thighs and wings are a better option. All the meats, especially chicken is high in nutrients and proteins. In order to get its proper nutrition, you should have meat once a week.

**Tomatoes -** Though counted as vegetables, tomatoes are actually fruits with only 4% carbs. In a big tomato, you will only find 7 grams of carbs. They are also high in potassium and vitamin C and are great for summer.

**Olives -** Olives only have 6% that is 2 grams per ounces of carbs. It is high in iron and copper and also provides Vitamin E to your body.

Other low carb foods you can adjust to your diet are full-fat yogurt, carrots, boiled eggs but not more than two. Include various veggies in your omelet at breakfast to make it healthy and low carb. In fruits, you can have apples, oranges, strawberries, pears. If you are interested in eating a dairy product then you can have cheese buttercream. Eggs are low in carbs and are a source of Omega 3, so you can eat it daily. You can have all kinds of meat - chicken, pork, lamb, etc. Most of the vegetables are low in carbs with lots of benefits - cabbage, broccoli, carrot, spinach, lady's finger but don't eat potatoes. It does more harm than good to your body.

Other than this you can include a lot of things in your low carb ration like olive oil, sour cream, nuts, blueberry, butter, coconut, fresh vegetables, sea salt, garlic. You can also consume dark chocolates and dry wine at long gaps. Make sure your wine has no added sugar.

# KETO DIETING? HERE ARE 10 FOODS YOU MUST HAVE IN YOUR KITCHEN

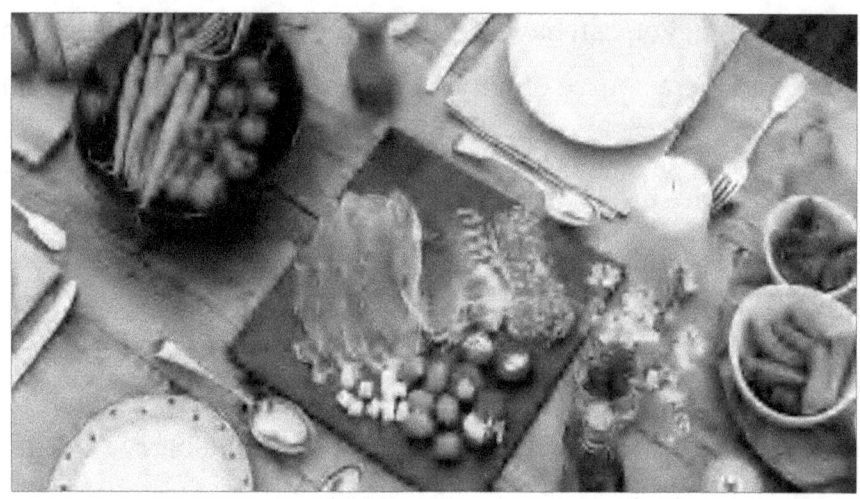

The ketogenic diet is a very successful weight-loss program. It utilizes high fat and low carbohydrate ingredients in order to burn fat instead of glucose. Many people are familiar with the Atkins diet, but the keto plan restricts carbs even more.

Because we are surrounded by fast food restaurants and processed meals, it can be a challenge to avoid carb-rich foods, but proper planning can help.

Plan menus and snacks at least a week ahead of time, so you aren't caught with only high carb meal choices. Research keto recipes online; there are quite a few good ones to choose from.

Immerse yourself in the keto lifestyle, find your favorite recipes, and stick with them.

There are a few items that are staples of a keto diet. Be sure to have these items on hand:

1. Eggs - Used in omelets, quiches (yes, heavy cream is legal on keto!), hard boiled as a snack, low carb pizza crust, and more; if you like eggs, you have a great chance of success on this diet

2. Bacon - Do I need a reason? breakfast, salad garnish, burger topper, BLT's (no bread of course; try a BLT in a bowl, tossed in mayo)

3. Cream cheese - Dozens of recipes, pizza crusts, main dishes, desserts

4. Shredded cheese - Sprinkle over taco meat in a bowl, made into tortilla chips in the microwave, salad toppers, low-carb pizza and enchiladas

5. Lots of romaine and spinach - Fill up on the green veggies; have plenty on hand for a quick salad when hunger pangs hit

6. EZ-Sweetz liquid sweetener - Use a couple of drops in place of sugar; this artificial sweetener is the most natural and easiest to use that I've found

7. Cauliflower - Fresh or frozen bags you can eat this low-carb veggie by itself, tossed in olive oil and baked, mashed in fake potatoes, chopped/shredded and used in place of rice under main dishes, in low-carb and keto pizza crusts, and much more

8. Frozen chicken tenders - Have a large bag on hand; thaw quickly and grill, saute, mix with veggies and top with garlic sauce in a low carb flatbread, use in Chicken piccata, chicken alfredo, tacos, enchiladas, Indian Butter chicken, and more

9. Ground beef - Make a big burger and top with all sorts of things from cheese, to sauteed mushrooms, to grilled onions... or crumble and cook with taco seasoning and use in provolone cheese taco shells; throw in a dish with lettuce, avocado, cheese, sour cream for a tortilla-less taco salad

10. Almonds (plain or flavored) - these are a tasty and healthy snack; however, be sure to count them as you eat, because the carbs DO add up. Flavors include habanero, coconut, salt and vinegar and more.

The keto plan is a versatile and interesting way to lose weight, with lots of delicious food choices. Keep these 10 items stocked in your fridge, freezer, and larder, and you'll be ready to throw together some delicious keto meals and snacks at a moment's notice

# FOODS TO AVOID WHEN USING A KETOGENIC DIET FOR WEIGHT LOSS

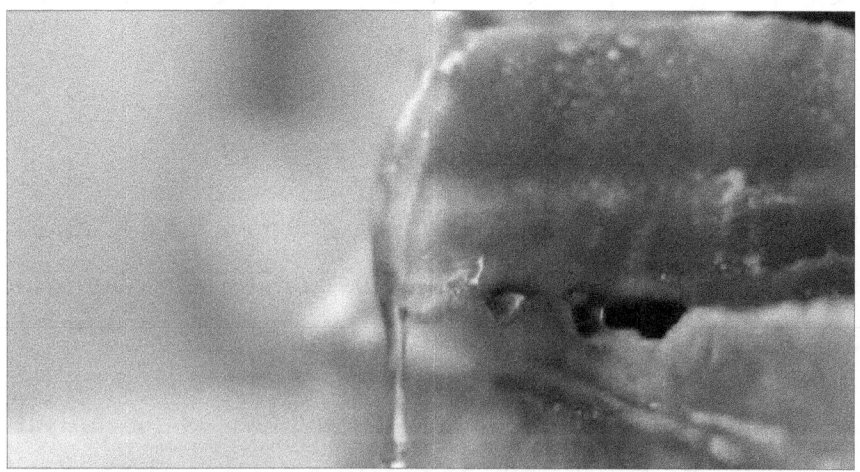

It is important to know the kinds of food you should avoid in order to remain in an optimal state of ketosis. The essence of reducing carbohydrates in a ketogenic diet is simply to induce the state of ketosis.

Proteins and fat are therefore regulated as a way of stopping the body from adapting to these dietary modifications.

## *Fats*

The ketogenic diet by nature encourages the consumption of healthy fats. This serves as the main energy for the body during the state of ketosis.

Most ketogenic diets consume about 60 to 80% of the daily calorie intake from fats. However, this value is dependent on the intended purpose of the diet. In the treatment of epilepsy, 90% of the daily calorie intake comes exclusively from fats.

Below are a few tips on choosing the best type of fats to include in your ketogenic diet.

## Polyunsaturated (PUFAs) Omega-6 Fats

When consumed in large amounts, omega-6 fatty acids can cause inflammation in the body. This can just be as damaging as the increase in sugar consumption.

Also, seed or nut-based oil should be avoided as they are also high in omega-6 that can have an inflammatory effect.

Some of the polyunsaturated fatty acids and nut-based oil to avoid include:

Canola oil, Corn oil, Cottonseed oil, Flax oil, Grapeseed oil, Peanut oil, Safflower oil, Sesame oil, Soybean oil, Sunflower oil, Vegetable oil, Walnut oil

## Hydrogenated and Trans Fats

Trans fat is the most inflammatory of all fats. Several studies have noted that foods containing trans fats increase the risk of developing heart disease and cancer.

Also, avoid mayonnaise and commercial salad dressing and if unavoidable, check their carbohydrate content and include in it your carbohydrate counts.

## Proteins

The choice of your proteins in a ketogenic diet is very important. Your protein can affect the diet over the course of time. Animals that have been treated with steroids and antibiotics have the potential to cause health problems.

It is always best to purchase grass-fed, organic and free-range humanely raised animals. Avoid hormone-fed animals, especially with rBST.

Also, when buying processed meat products, you should check the carbohydrate content as they might have been added through the extenders and fillers used. You need to also avoid meats that have been cured with sugar or honey.

## Carbohydrates

Reduction of carbohydrate food intake is the main focus of ketogenic diets. However, the level of restriction of carbohydrate intake is mostly based on the individual's activity level and metabolic rate.

Keeping your carbohydrate intake to less than 30 grams a day will help you to remain in ketosis. However, individuals that have a healthy metabolism and those with higher metabolic rates (such as athletes) can afford to eat as much as 50 grams of carbohydrate daily.

Those with metabolic issues (such as Type 2 Diabetes) and sedentary persons need to stay at fewer than 20 grams of carbohydrate per day. Another factor might also be the purpose of the ketogenic diet.

Some of the common carbohydrates to avoid include the following grains and grain products:

Amaranth, Barley, Bread crumbs, Bread, Buckwheat, Bulgur, Cakes, Cookies, Corn chips, Cornbread, Cornmeal, Crackers, Grits, Kashi, Muffins, Oatmeal, Oats, Pancakes, Pasta, Pies,

Polenta, Popcorn, Pretzels, Quinoa, Rice, Rolls, Rye, Sorghum, Spelt, Tarts, Tortillas, Triticale, Waffles, Wheat

## *Vegetables*

Vegetables are the main carbohydrate sources in a ketogenic diet. Also, a lot of vegetables that grow underground are starchy and contain a lot of carbohydrates.

You should limit your consumption of Brussels sprout, green beans and pumpkin as the carbs can add up quickly.

However, you should avoid the following vegetables:

Carrots, Corn, Green peas, Leeks, Parsnips, Potatoes, Squash, Sweet potatoes, Yams, Yuca **Tropical Fruits**

Avoid most tropical fruits including mango, papaya, and pineapple as they are usually high carbohydrates. Also, avoid 100 percent fresh juice since most of them are often high in sugars.

## *Sugars and Sweeteners*

Sugar is a very rich source of glucose and must, therefore, be avoided. Also, sugar is known in forms like brown sugar, white, castor and icing sugar. Sugar can also be an ingredient in processed foods.

Barley malt, Beet sugar, Brown sugar, cane juice, Cane syrup, Caramel, Carob syrup, Coconut sugar, Corn syrup, Date sugar, Fruit juice concentrate, Fruit syrups, Malt syrup, Maltose, Maple syrup, Molasses, Panela, Panocha, Rice Syrup, Sorghum, Tapioca syrup, Treacle, Turbinado sugar, White sugar.

# MANAGING WEIGHT LOSS

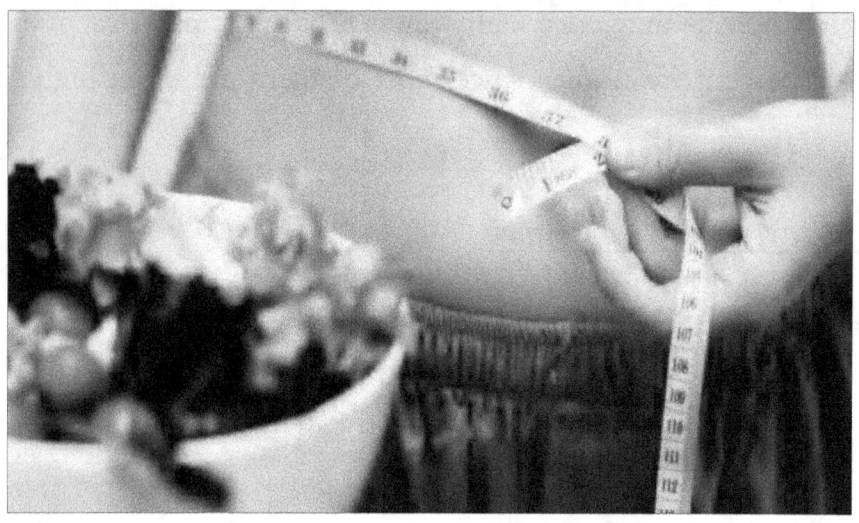

It is a well-known fact that obesity is now an epidemic in America. Almost 40% of Americans including children are overweight, and most people have tried many different diet plans with varying success.

Before embarking on a weight loss program, it is important to recognize that occasionally, there may be a medical condition that may be responsible for weight gain. Conditions affecting the metabolism such as hypothyroidism, Cushing's syndrome, polycystic ovary syndrome as well as some medications such as corticosteroids, cyproheptadine, lithium, tranquilizers, phenothiazines, and tricyclic antidepressants can cause weight gain

However, for most people, the reason for weight gain is too many calories consumed and not enough exercise! The question is, how to curb your appetite and in such a situation. Understanding the causes of hunger can go a long way in managing hunger and weight loss.

## *Understanding Cause of Hunger*

Sugar intake affects hunger. Insulin levels in the blood have a direct impact on hunger. The primary role of insulin is to regulate the fuel in the body by transporting glucose from the blood into the cells. Higher the amount of insulin circulating in the blood, faster it will store the sugar in the cells as fat, if the sugar, that is, energy, is not used in activities such as work or exercise thus lowering the sugar level in the blood, making you hungry and craving for sweets.

## *Managing Weight Loss*

Cut back on sugar in all of its forms; soda, ice cream, cake, dessert, and chocolate. Sugar triggers the appetite soon after consumption by raising the blood sugar levels. The rapid absorption of sucrose causes a sudden spurt of insulin, which leads to a rapid dip in the blood sugar levels and causes hunger.

Modify your diet. Add banana, peanuts, almonds, milk, cheese, egg yolk, chicken and lamb to your diet. These foods contain amino acid tryptophan which is responsible for suppressing appetite. It helps in the formation of a brain chemical serotonin, which signals the brain to transmit "I am full" messages thereby reducing your appetite.

According to some researchers, a bowl of chicken soup or a glass of lime juice taken about half an hour before a meal stimulates the level of your hormone called CCK (Cholecystokinin) thereby suppressing your appetite. Black coffee or tea also raises your CCK level.

Stress also has an important role in appetite control. During a stressful situation, the bloodstream is flooded with glucose and you do not think of food but later blood sugar drops and you feel very hungry.

Exercise helps reduce hunger by releasing chemicals such as endorphins that diminish hunger and helps alleviate anxiety and depression. Exercise also helps burn extra calories. Endorphin is also responsible for giving you the feeling of well being.

Yoga helps reduce hunger as well. A study undertaken in 10 Type II diabetic patients and published in the Journal of the Association of Physicians of India (JAPI) by Dr. Vijay Vishwanathan, Dr. P. T Chacko, and others have shown how performing Yogasanas (various routines of Yoga) can be considered not as an adjunct but as an alternative method of treating diabetes. The unexpected results were improved insulin sensitivity in the Yogasanas group.

Take dietary supplements. Adding nutritional supplements to your diet daily helps balance your body's needs for necessary nutrients. Supplements such as fish oil supplements, 5HTP, 7 Keto, Guggulipid, Chromium picolinate, Gymnema Silvestre and Green Tea can help manage your weight loss. Supplement websites or stores carry these supplements in Weight Management or Weight Loss categories or section.

# HEALTHY WEIGHT LOSS -
# MAINTAINING A HEAL WEIGHT LOSS

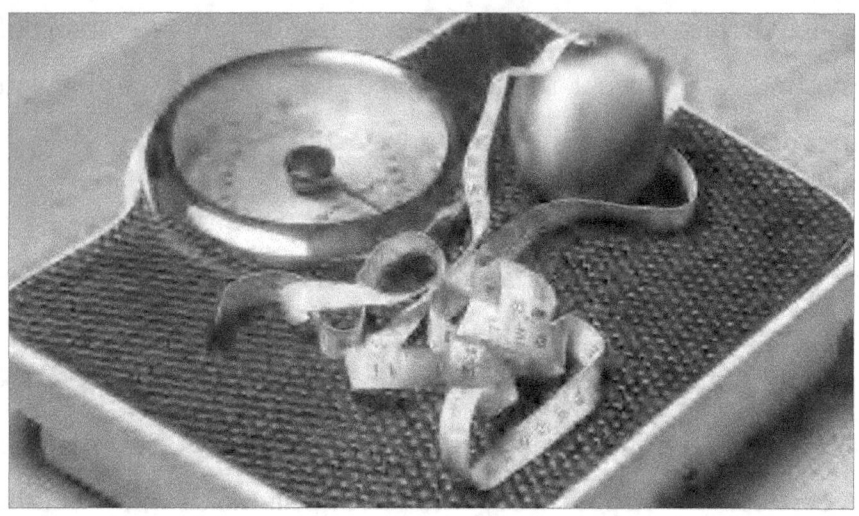

While the desire to shed the pounds quickly is definitely strong, it's incredibly important that throughout your quest you try and maintain a healthy weight loss. Those individuals who choose to go on crash diets will lose weight, however not only is the weight loss not likely to stay off, but these crash diets are also going to severely affect their health status and metabolism.

Whenever you see a diet out there promising to help you lose ten or more pounds a week, automatic red flags should be raised on not only the safety of this approach but also how well it will actually work.

If the truth was told, even if you ate absolutely nothing for an entire week straight, you still would not lose 10 pounds of pure fat a week, so claims such as these are completely unrealistic. You may lose a good amount of water weight - there's no doubting that, and it could amount to ten pounds when combined with muscle glycogen losses as well, but rest assured, once you come off your starvation fast, that weight will come rushing back on to your body.

Therefore, here are some simple tips you need to keep in mind so you can maintain a healthy weight loss.

## *Always Include A Variety of Vegetables*

The largest portion of most diets will usually be vegetables and possibly fruits (depending on the individual plan). If you're currently on a weight loss plan that restricts the amount of product you're able to eat, you want to rethink that plan.

Vegetables are pretty much 'free foods' as far as calories are concerned (with the exception of possibly corn, peas, and potatoes), so you should be able to eat them to your heart's content.

Not only that but they are loaded with potassium, which will help you maintain your energy for exercise.

## Don't Eliminate Carbs Entirely

While low-carb diets definitely are all the rage right now, completely eliminating carbohydrates from your daily diet is a big mistake.

Unless you are following a very specific keto plan set-up, which is an ultra low-carb diet but actually changes the type of fuel your body runs off of, you need carbohydrates to function.

You may be able to cut them out for three to four days, but it's almost guaranteed that after that, you're going to be craving carbohydrates so strongly that it becomes almost impossible not to include some in your diet.

A better approach is using a more moderate carb intake, so you both maintain your energy levels and keeping sanity in check.

Carbohydrates do not limit your ability to lose weight if the weight loss plan is set up properly.

## Plan For Cheat Days To Maintain a Healthy Weight Loss

Finally, the last thing you must consider is your psychological relationship with food. When we diet, we often start playing mind games with ourselves and some of us actually become somewhat 'fearful' in a sense of certain foods.

You really must watch this because, in the long run, it can set you up for emotional eating problems associated with binging or other eating disorders down the road.

If you plan and schedule in cheat meals and days into your diet, you will help yourself maintain a good relationship with food and you will see that realistically, one meal off your diet is not going to undo all the hard work you've put in.

You can most definitely still have great results with your weight loss plan when including cheat meals and cheat days.

So, be sure you keep these points in mind so you can maintain a healthy weight loss. Taking short-cuts, eliminating too many foods, and trying to starve yourself thin will all backfire in the end, so it's much better to just avoid this in the first place.

# HOW THE KETOGENIC DIET WORKS IN WEIGHT LOSS

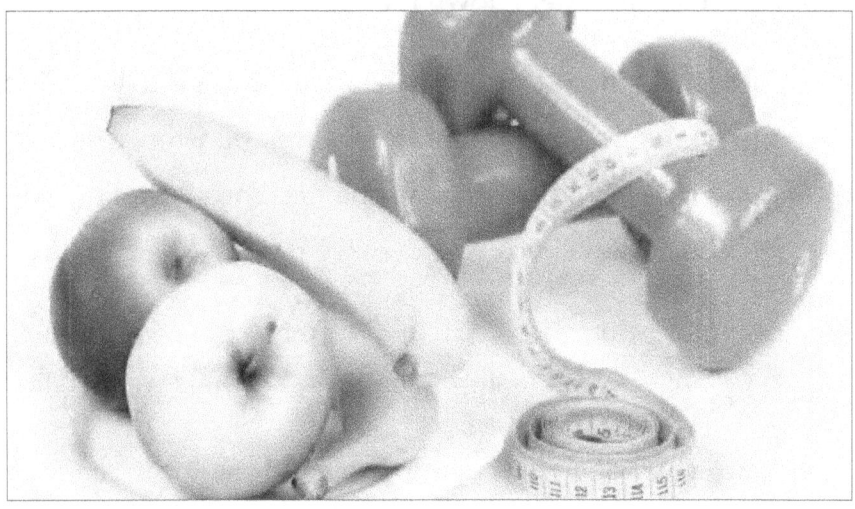

Ketogenic diets force the body to enter into a state called ketosis. The body generally makes use of carbohydrate as its primary source of energy. This owes to the fact that carbohydrates are the easiest for the body to absorb.

However, should the body run out of carbohydrates, it reverts to making use of fats and protein for its energy production. Essentially, the body has a sort of energy hierarchy which it follows.

Firstly, the body is programmed to use carbohydrate as energy fuel when it is available. Secondly, it will revert to using fats as an alternative in the absence of an adequate supply of carbohydrate.

Lastly, the body will turn to proteins for its energy provision in when there is an extreme depletion of its carbohydrate and fat stores. However, breaking down proteins for energy provision leads to a general loss of lean muscle mass.

The ketogenic diet does not fully depend on the calories in, calories out model. This is because of the composition of those calories matters due to the hormonal response of the body to different macronutrients.

However, there are two schools of thought in the keto community. While one believes that the amount of calories and fat consumption does not matter, the other contends that calories and fat do matter.

When using a ketogenic diet, you are trying to find a balance point. While calories matter, the composition of those calories also counts. In a ketogenic diet, the most important factor of the composition of those calories is the balance of fat, protein, and carbohydrates and how each affects insulin levels.

This balance is very important because any rise in insulin will stop lipolysis. Therefore, you need to eat foods that will create the smallest rise in insulin. This will help to keep your body in the state of burning stored body fat for fuel - lipolysis.

The body can normally go into a ketosis state by itself. This is often the case when you are in a fasting state such as when you are sleeping. In this state, the body tends to burn fats for energy while the body carries out its repairs and growth while you sleep.

Carbohydrates generally make up most of the calories in a regular meal. Also, the body is inclined to make use of the carbohydrate as energy as it is more easily absorbable. The proteins and fats in the diet are thus more likely to be stored.

However, in a ketogenic diet, most of the calories come from fats rather than carbohydrates. Since ketogenic diets have a low amount of carbohydrates, they are immediately used up. The low carbohydrate level causes an apparent shortage of energy fuel for the body.

As a result of this seeming shortage, the body resorts to its stored fat content. It makes a shift from a carbohydrate-consumer to a fat-burner. The body, however, does not make use of the fats in the recently ingested meal but rather stores them up for the next round of ketosis.

As the body gets more familiar to burning fat for energy, fats in an ingested meal become used up with little left for storage.

This is why the ketogenic diet uses a high amount of fat consumption so that the body can have enough for energy production and also still be able to store some fat. The body needs to be able to store some fat otherwise it will start breaking down its protein stores in muscles during the ketosis period.

In fasting periods - such as during ketosis, in between meals and during sleep - the body still needs a constant supply of energy. You have these periods in your normal day and therefore you need to consume enough amounts of fat for your body to use as energy.

If there are no adequate amounts of stored fat, the proteins contained in your muscle become the next option for the body to use as energy. It is therefore important to eat enough to avoid this scenario from taking place.

The main goal of a ketogenic diet is to mimic the state of starvation in the body. Ketogenic diets deprive the body of its preferred immediate and easily convertible carbohydrates by restricting and severely cutting back on carbohydrate intake. This situation forces it into a fat burning mode for energy production.

# KETOGENIC DIETS AND WEIGHT LOSS AND BODYBUILDING

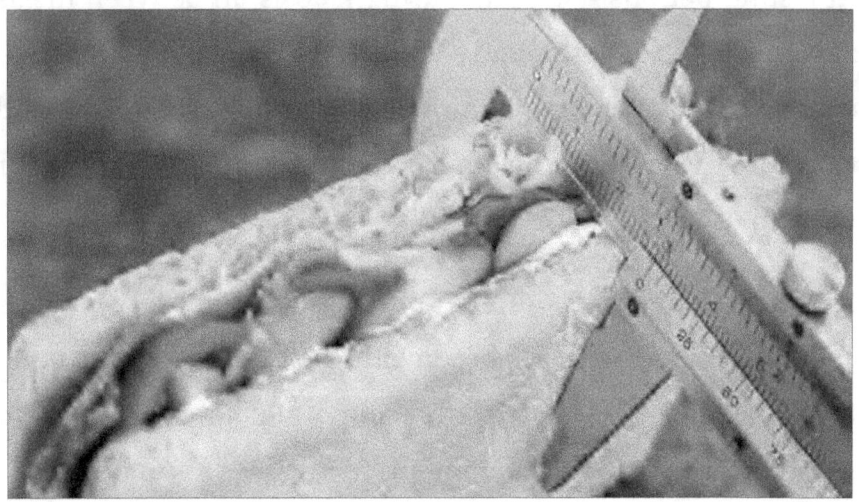

People always want to know what the best diet is or what they can do to lose fat faster. Truthfully, most people have no clue what they are getting themselves into. While a ketogenic diet may work better than a low carb diet, people should be ready for them.

First off, a ketogenic diet is one where there are no carbs. Without carbohydrates, the body turns to burn fat as the primary fuel source. Since this is happening the body can tap into stored body fat for energy and we can end up leaner. Well while that is possible we need to look at what may happen.

For starters, your energy will be drained. Without carbohydrates, your body won't know what energy source to turn to for a few days so you may experience feelings of weakness while you train or until your body becomes adapted at using fat. While this isn't a bad thing you must understand that you have to change your training intensity. There's no way that you can keep training with super high volume while you use one of these diets.

The next thing that you have to understand about using a ketogenic diet for weight loss or bodybuilding is that you need to eat more protein then normal. Since you don't have carbs, and carbs are protein sparing, you need to consume more protein so you don't lose muscle tissue. So make sure that you are eating at least 6 meals per day with a serving of protein coming to every meal.

Then you have to make sure that you are getting enough fiber. Look to consume fiber from various sources such as green vegetables and fiber powder or pills like a physillum husk. Now you need to add some healthily nutritional supplements since you want to make sure that you do your best to burn fat on these keto diets for weight loss and bodybuilding. First, make sure you consume healthy fats like omega-3 fish oils, CLA, and gla. These fats will help to burn more body fat. Then you want to purchase a good branch chain amino acid powder as bcaa's help to retain muscle mass and prevent muscle breakdown.

So in conclusion, a ketogenic diet may be the best for weight loss or bodybuilding but you need to make sure you are eating enough and taking in the right nutrients or you'll lose too much muscle mass.

# LOSING WEIGHT FACTORS TO CONSIDER

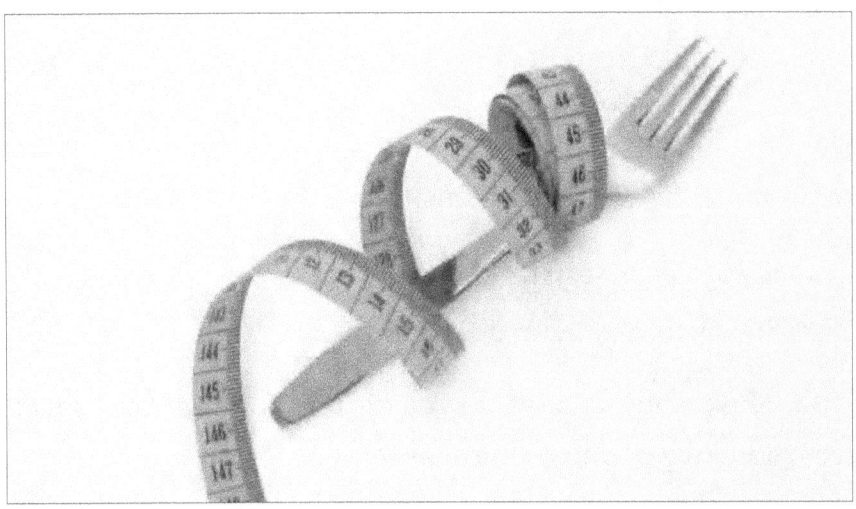

There are many reasons why being overweight is bad for your health. It can, for example, cause or aggravate type 2 diabetes. Obesity is also a risk factor for heart disease and other cardiovascular problems.

## *So what do you have to do to lose weight?*

Eat less and move more is the trite answer usually received by someone who is overweight.

Of course, you can lose weight by reducing the food you eat (energy intake) or increasing the amount of exercise you get (energy output).

But the problem of effective weight-loss is much more complex than simply changing the balance between the calories you consume and the calories you expend in your daily activities.

The search for an effective weight-loss formula requires answers to these four questions:

- Does genetics play a role in your weight problems and, if so, what can you do about it?

- How many calories do you need to cut from your diet to lose one pound or kilogram?

- What are the best types of foods (carbs, fats or proteins) to cut for losing weight? Is exercise much good in helping you lose weight or for keeping weight off?

## _How genes affect your weight_

Many people do their utmost to lose weight without much success. In particular, once they have lost a few kilos, they find it extremely difficult to keep their weight down... it just rises back up again.

This suggests that the problem is genetic.

In fact, more than 30 genes have been linked to obesity. The one with the strongest link is the fat mass and obesity associated gene (FTO).

The obesity-risk variant of the FTO gene affects one in six of the population. Studies suggest that persons who have this gene are 70% more likely to become obese.

According to research published in the UK in 2013 in the Journal of Clinical Investigation, people with this gene have higher levels of the ghrelin, the hunger hormone, in their blood. This means they start to feel hungry again soon after eating a meal.

In addition, real-time brain imaging shows that the FTO gene variation changes the way the brain responds to ghrelin and images of food in the regions of the brain linked to the control of eating and reward.

These findings explain why people with the obesity-risk variant of the FTO gene eat more and prefer higher calorie foods... even before they become overweight... compared with those with the low-risk version of the gene.

The FTO gene is not the only genetic cause of obesity, which is likely to be due to the sum of several genes working together.

If you have these 'bad' genes, however, you are not necessarily destined to become overweight... but you are more likely to end up obese if you over-eat.

Having these genes also means that you will need to exercise greater discipline over your diet throughout your life, especially when you have managed to shed a few pounds and want to keep them off.

## *How many calories should you cut to lose weight?*

The big question for dieters has always been... how many calories do I need to cut out of my diet in order to reduce my weight by a set amount, eg one pound or kilogram?

Once upon a time, there was a clear-cut answer to this question.

In 1958 Max Wishnofsky, a New York doctor, wrote a paper that summed up everything known at that time about how calories are stored in our bodies. He concluded that, if your weight is being held steady, it would take a deficit of 3,500 calories to lose one pound (454 grams) in weight.

You could create the calorie deficit either by eating less or exercising more (to use up more calories).

For example, if your weight is holding steady on a diet of 2,000 calories a day and you reduce your intake to 1,500 calories a day, you will lose one pound (nearly half a kilo) in one week, ie 52 pounds or 24kg a year.

Alternatively, you could burn an extra 500 calories a day (through exercise) to lose the same amounts of weight over the same time periods.

For years, the Wishnofsky rule was accepted as a verified fact. It underpinned a wide variety of diets.

The only problem is that the rule is wrong. It fails to take into account the changes in metabolism that take place when you go on a weight-reducing diet.

The Wishnofsky rule actually works initially. But after a week or two, your weight reaches its minimal level, much to the frustration of myriads of dieters, as your metabolism adjusts to the decrease in your body mass and your reduced intake of food.

Until recently there was no way to predict how consuming fewer calories affects the rate at which you will lose weight, especially when your goal is to lose more than just a few pounds or kilograms.

There are now, however, new complex weight-loss formulas that factor in the drop in metabolic rate that occurs over time as body mass decreases. One example is the Body Weight

Planner from the National Institute of Diabetes and Kidney and Digestive Diseases in the USA.

## What types of foods should you cut to lose weight?

Should you reduce your calories from your fat, carbohydrate or protein intakes? Which will help you lose weight faster?

The numbers of calories in one gram of each of the basic food types are as follows:

- Fat... 9 calories per gram

- Drinking Alcohol... 7 calories per gram

- Proteins... 4 calories per gram

- Carbohydrates... 4 calories per gram

- Dietary Fibre... 2 calories per gram

As fats contain more than twice as many calories as carbs and proteins, reducing the fats you eat will work twice as quickly as a reduction in either of the other two types of foods, gram for gram.

This is why diets that concentrate on reducing the fat you eat, such as the Beating Diabetes Diet and the Mediterranean Diet are effective in reducing weight.

But if you want to cut your calorie intake by a fixed amount a day (say 500 calories) will it make any difference as to which type of food you cut down on?

For example, will it make any difference to the amount of weight you lose if you cut 55.6 grams of fat (500 calories) or 125g of carbs (500 calories) or 125g of protein (500 calories) from your diet?

The answer is that there is little difference in the number of weight people lose whether they cut their calories from carbs or fat.

But calories from proteins are different... according to researchers, high-protein diets tend to increase the number of calories you burn. Why this is so is not clear.

However, when people lose weight they lose muscle as well as fat. The more muscle you lose the more your metabolism slows down which reduces the rate at which you lose weight.

Because it preserves muscle, a protein-based diet may reduce the rate at which your metabolism slows down.

The problem is that, if you eat too much protein, you could end up damaging your kidneys. The generally accepted recommendation is that you limit your protein intake to a maximum of 35% of your total daily intake of calories.

So, provided you don't eat too much protein, it is best to reduce weight by cutting down on fats (for the sake of your heart, etc) and refined carbs that spike blood glucose levels (especially if you have diabetes).

Does exercise help you lose weight or keep it off?

Cutting down on the food you eat is the best way to lose weight. Exercise is less important, at least in the initial stages.

Exercising when you are trying to lose weight can be tricky. It burns calories for sure but not nearly as many as not eating those calories in the first place.

And exercise increases your appetite, so it is easy to eat back on all the calories you burn during an intense workout.

The recommendation, when you are cutting your food intake to lose weight, is to focus on moderate physical activities such as gardening or brisk walking, rather than going to the gym.

But once you have shred those extra pounds and are down to your ideal weight, exercise becomes important for maintaining your weight at its new healthier level.

Researchers have found that most people who lose weight and manage to keep it off for at least a year exercise regularly for up to an hour every day.

# LOSE WEIGHT FAST THANKS TO A KETOGENIC TYPE OF DIET

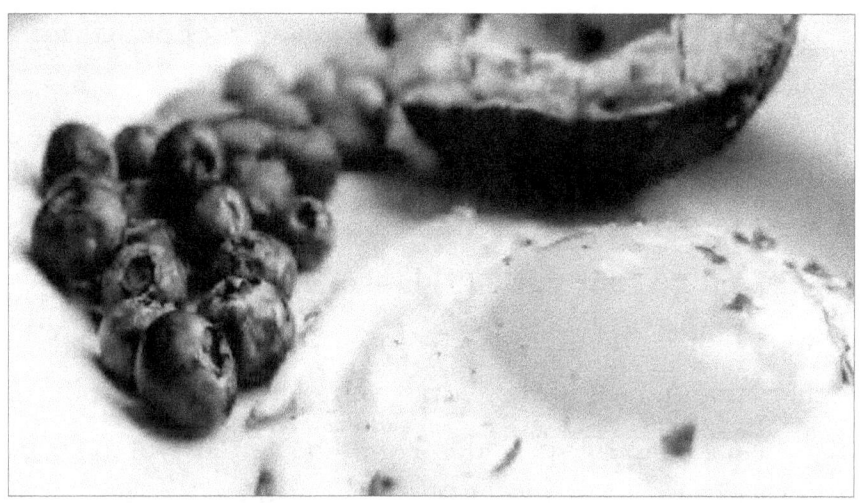

The ketogenic diet is a diet based on a process called ketosis. It is a specific state of the body, which is characterized by an elevated level of ketones in the blood, which occurs due to the conversion of fats into fatty acids and ketones. This occurs when the body gets only very small amounts of carbohydrates over a certain period of time. When you start with this type of diet, your body goes through several changes. After 24-48 hours since the beginning of this diet, the body starts to use ketones in order to use the energy stored in fat cells more efficiently. In other words, the primary source of energy becomes fat (fatty acids), instead of carbohydrates (glucose).

Because of that, during ketosis, it is not a problem to eat food with higher amounts of fat than would otherwise seem reasonable. This way the body is rapidly losing weight (specifically fat). In addition, the loss of muscle tissue (proteins) is minimal, since the vast majority of food consumed during ketosis, also contains relatively large amounts of proteins that are good for your muscles.

Although ketosis is the basis of the ketogenic type of diet, in its strictest form it doesn't need to be kept for long. The state of ketosis can be held up until the body weight is just a few pounds higher than the one that is desired. Then foods with higher amounts of carbohydrates are gradually introduced (rice, beans...). In this period, it would be very useful to keep a food intake diary in which daily amounts of taken carbs would be noted. That way you can find the maximum amount of daily carbs that still allows you not to gain weight. Once you discover this parameter, you will no longer have overweight related problems, because until that moment you will certainly learn to take account of calories and amounts of carbs, proteins, and fats that you consume daily. That way you will get to know your body better, in terms of the maximum "allowable" daily intake. Because of that, we could say that the ketogenic diet is, in a way, a procedure for learning habits that will ensure that you never return to the old potentially problematic overweight levels.

There are many types of ketogenic diets that can be found on the internet or in other sources, but they all have in common one basic principle - intake of high amounts of proteins and fats, and minimal amounts of carbohydrates. Which exact diet you will choose, isn't as important, as long as it will allow you to enter ketosis, which is the basis of the biological mechanism that will help you lose weight efficiently.

# LOW-CARB AND KETO DIET FAST FOOD MENU CHOICES: HOW TO EAT SUCCESSFULLY AT RESTAURANTS

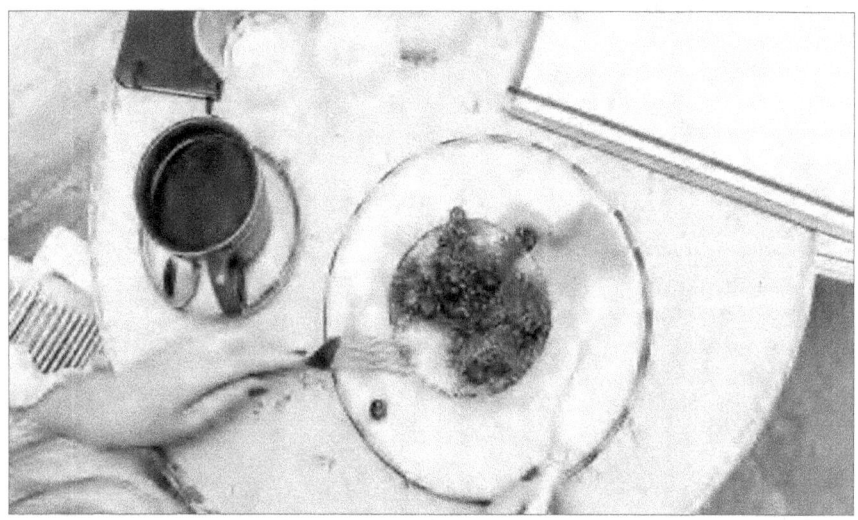

For those who eat low-carb or keto diets, there is almost always something you can eat in every fast food place or restaurant. Plan ahead. Before entering a restaurant, check out their menu and nutrition information online at home or using your smartphone. It's always good to know the safe options before being tempted by menu items you shouldn't have on a low-carb diet.

In order to make it easier to find a quick keto-friendly option, a list of several restaurants and fast food places and those items found to be the lowest carb (and most emotionally satisfying) choices. These are not all perfect options, but when you're stuck with no other choices due to time or location constraints, they'll do in a pinch.

It's a huge help that fast-food places are required to post nutritional content. It gets easier to follow the keto plan every day. The carb count I'm listing is approximate and is NET grams.

In general, there is usually some salad option anywhere you are. At Burger joints, just remove the bun, and many places offer lettuce wraps instead. Chicken shouldn't have breading.

As a side note, it helps to have a knife and fork handy in your car or purse. Big, juicy burgers in tiny pieces of lettuce end up on the table - or in your lap. Small, flimsy fast-food plasticware also makes for difficult eating. Pull out your own sturdy utensils and enjoy!

Now for the food choices... here are some pretty obvious general rules to follow:

- Skip the bun or wrap
- Skip the pasta, potato, or rice

**Salads** - no croutons. Stick with low sugar dressing options - Caesar, Blue Cheese, Ranch, Chipotle. Look at the name which may give you a clue, things like "honey" in the honey dijon or "sweet" in the dressing name - these are usually not a good choice. Check the ingredient for items that are higher in carb content.

**Chicken** - Choose grilled or sauteed. Stay away from any chicken that is breaded.

**McDonald's** - opt for any burger (zero-g) or grilled chicken (2 g) without the bun and topped with cheese, mayo, mustard, onions, etc. No ketchup. Add a side salad (3g). The Caesar salad with grilled chicken or the bacon ranch salad with grilled chicken is 9g.

**Burger King** - same burger info as McDonald's: burger (zero-g) without the bun and topped with cheese, mayo, mustard, onions, etc. No ketchup. The tender grill chicken sandwich without the bun is 3g.

BEWARE - you might think the veggie burger is low, but it is 19g of carbs, so that's about a full day of carbs on keto. Add a side salad (3g). The tender grill chicken garden salad is 8g without dressing or croutons. The tender crisp chicken salad is not an option. Do not attempt.

BONUS - dessert!?! - the fresh apple fries are not fried and are 5g net carbs WITHOUT caramel sauce.

**Subway** - Probably should skip Subway if you can. The buns and wraps are all high in carbs. I guess you could just have them throw the ingredients in a wrapper sans bun, but that doesn't sound appealing. I have no info on what the carb count would be for each bunless sub, but you can probably figure it out - chicken or pepperoni is fine, but is "sweet onion" chicken okay? No idea. Stick to the salads, but realize you'll only get iceberg lettuce (4g).

**Carl's Junior and Hardees** - This chain offers "lettuce wraps" - your burger wrapped in a large piece of lettuce for easy low carb eating. (As I've said, I tried it and don't love it. I like to carry my own fork instead.) Bunless options - Six dollar burger (7g), 1/2 thick-burger (5g), charbroiled chicken club sandwich (7g/10g at Hardee's). Grilled chicken salad without croutons is 10g. The side salad is 3g.

**Jimmy John's** - The Dunwich - a sandwich wrapped in lettuce - fits the bill here. Meats are fine, just make sure the ingredients are not carb-rich. Wendy's - Again, you can get your burger in a lettuce wrap or a box. Any burger with toppings. Mayo has corn syrup and is 1g. The chicken grill fillet is 1 g. It can be ordered in the chicken club sandwich or the ultimate chicken grill sandwich. Best salads: chicken caesar (7g), blt chicken salad with grilled chicken. Side salads are 6g or 2g for Caesar.

**Pizza Hut and other pizza places** - It is possible to get used to eating pizza with no crust. You need to eat twice as much, but if there's a party or dinner out that you can't avoid at a pizza place, just slide the cheesy toppings off and eat the big messy pile of cheese and toppings. A side salad is a nice addition. Otherwise, just opt for making pizza at home with a low-carb crust.

**Mongolian Barbecue -** YES! Load up your bowl with chicken, shrimp, onion slices, and mushrooms, then top with the Asian black bean sauce. Beans have carbs, but this sauce label says 1 gram of carbs per ounce (each sauce is plainly labeled). Add a bit of garlic and wait for the griller to do his work. It goes without saying that you skip the appetizers, tortillas, and rice. Ask the wait staff not to bring them to the table.

**Italian Restaurants -** These take a little cunning, but they can be conquered! Ideas: how about chicken Marsala in an Italian place? Make sure it doesn't come with pasta. Substitute broccoli or some other keto-friendly side dish - or a big salad. Chicken piccata is also a possibility.

Mexican and Chinese restaurants are the most difficult because any low carb option is not the reason to go to the restaurant in the first place. At a Mexican restaurant, you can get a large burrito with no beans and spread the soft tortilla out like a plate. Eat the inner ingredients and toss the tortilla.

If you MUST go to a Chinese buffet, you can find options, but they probably aren't going to be your favorite General Tso's. How about the salad bar choices? Eggs? The insides of eggrolls and ate the insides only of crab rangoons. Unfortunately, these ideas leave quite a pile of discarded shells and deep fried exterior pieces on your plate and make it look like you really waste food.

**Wings anywhere** - Standard buffalo sauce is usually OK as well as garlic Parmesan

Convenience stores can be a good option, too! 7-11 has packs of hard boiled eggs, cheese slabs, slim jims, almonds, and pork rinds. Pork rinds come in a barbecue flavor and they're ZERO carbs.

Remember, whatever you choose, hold the bread, potatoes, rice, noodles, fries, and tortillas. And watch out for the possibility of corn starch, bread crumbs, and other fillers. With proper planning and a good attitude, you can find healthy keto and low-carb options when dining out and stick to your successful keto diet plan.

# LOW CARBOHYDRATE NUTRITION
# WHAT THEY HAVE IN COMMON

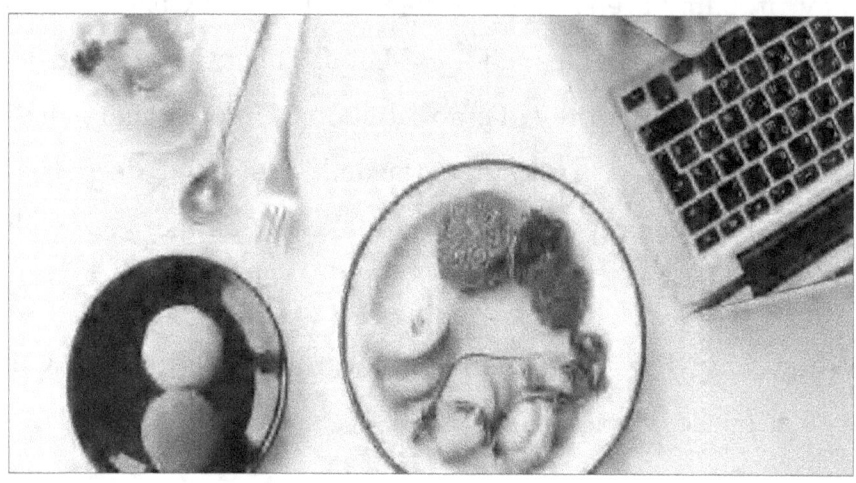

In recent years, many new types of nutrition have shown up, many of which are related to a state called ketosis. In this state, your body doesn't use carbohydrates anymore as the primary source of energy, but instead it uses your own body fat, and the fats that you take with your food. The state of ketosis is usually entered by going on a so-called, ketogenic type of diet, where you mostly eat food rich with proteins and fats (remember, you will burn that fat fast, so it's not a problem), but with very little or none carbohydrates. There are many ketogenic diets that can be found, either online, or from other sources, but here we will mention something that most of them have in common - nutrition with low carb content.

There are basically four different types of meals that can be prepared on these kinds of diets. Those are meals based on cheese, meals based on eggs, meals based on fish, and meals based on meat. All four of the basic ingredients that are mentioned here have the same property - they are rich in proteins and fats but have a low content of carbohydrates which is exactly what we want when being on a ketogenic diet or when we want to enter ketosis. Fresh cheese (quark), eggs, tuna, bacon, mayonnaise, roasted sausages, different types of omelets - these are just some of the many things you can eat on this type of diet.

That may sound like a great diet to be on, but it isn't really easy to be on this type of diet for longer periods of time (and it is not really advisable), so it is good (and necessary, because of the vitamins, fibers, and minerals you will get from vegetables) to also include some vegetables, but only those with a low content of carbohydrates, like: cabbage, green salad (lettuce), cucumbers and other similar vegetables. Other types of vegetables, like potatoes, beans, and peas should be avoided because they have a relatively high content of carbohydrates.

You may also wish to occasionally eat something sweet for a change. This may be a bit tricky, because you will have to use artificial sweeteners, but there are many products made for people with diabetes, that contain no sugar, and can thereby also be used by people that are on a ketogenic diet.

# KETO MEAL PLAN

## PROT- PACKED

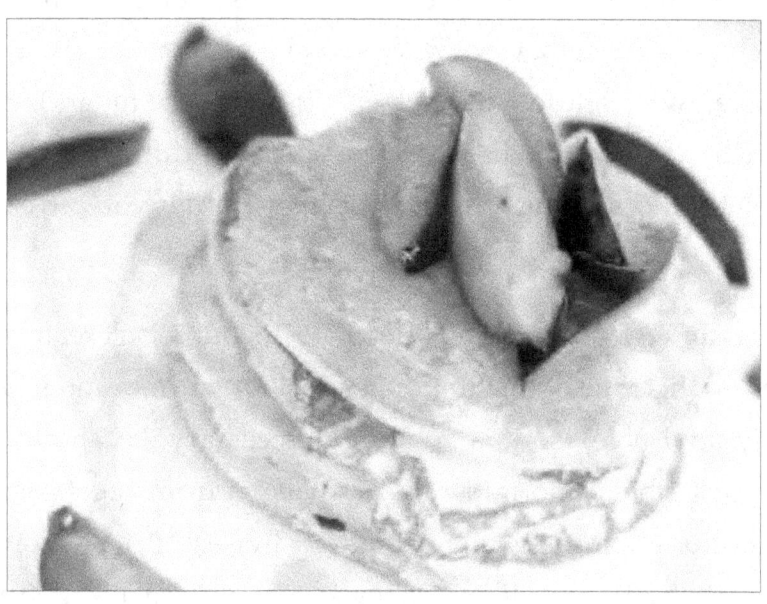

**Servings**: 4

If you're beginning a keto diet, it's important to understand how to build your meals so you eat a healthy balance of carbohydrates, fats, and protein. Below are quick and easy to start keto meal plan.

# WEEK ONE

## MONDAY BREAKFAST

### Ingredients

- 2 scoops vanilla protein powder

- 2 tsp baking powder

- 1 pinch of salt

- tbsp coconut flour

- medium eggs

- ¼ tsp vanilla extract

- 4 tbsp softened butter

- tbsp heavy cream

- tbsp syrup

### Directions:

1. Mix dry ingredients in a bowl then set aside.

2. Mix wet ingredients. Add a pinch of salt if using unsalted butter.

3 . Create a well in the dry ingredients and pour in the wet ingredients, mixing well to evenly combine.

4 . Optional: Mix in extra ingredients such as berries, nuts, etc.

5 . Heat a flat pan and drizzle with cooking oil.

6 . Ladle a ¼ cup of batter into the pan for each pancake.

7 . Allow the pancake to cook until bubbles form on the surface, then flip.

8 . Cook another side for about one minute, then remove from heat and serve.

## Macros

- 37g fat ☐ 38g protein ☐ 1g carb
- 500 calories

# LUNCH

## ASIAN PUMPKIN

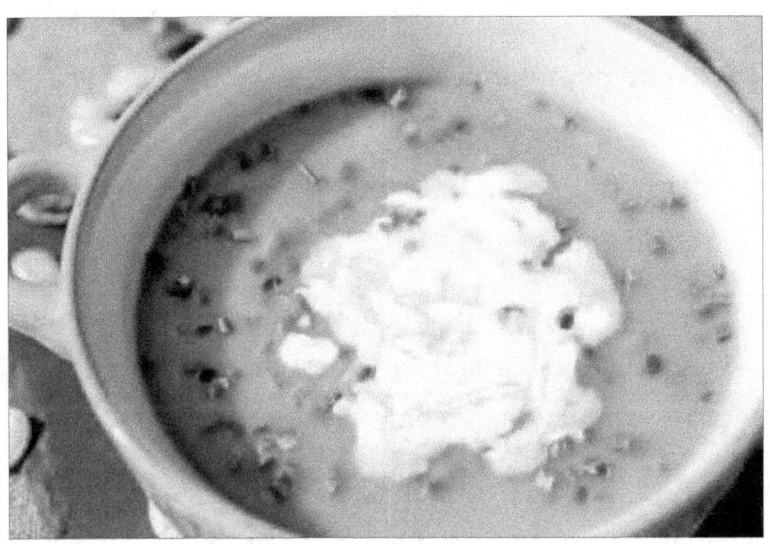

Servings: 4

## Ingredients

- 3 pounds pumpkin (the Japanese variety is recommended)

- 1/4 cup olive oil

- 1 teaspoon salt

- white onion, medium

- tablespoons butter (you may also use ghee)

- 2 cups heavy cream (coconut cream may be used instead)

- 1 tablespoon garlic powder

- 4 sprigs of rosemary

- 1/2 to 1 cup broth (you may use water if you prefer)

- 1/3 cup pumpkin seeds

## Directions:

1. Preheat your oven to 400°F.

2. Cut open the pumpkin and scrape out the pulp and seeds. Leave the skin on, and chop the pumpkin into cubes, about 2 inches on each side.

3. Spread the pieces out on a baking sheet and drizzle with olive oil. Season with a teaspoon of salt.

4. Place the baking sheet in the oven and bake for 40 minutes.

5. Chop the white onion finely. Melt some butter in a pan over low heat and cook until the pieces are translucent. Remove the pan from the heat.

6. Blend 2 cups of cream in a food processor until the consistency is light. This should take about 5 minutes.

7. Add the white onion, garlic powder, and rosemary into the blend and season to taste with some salt. Blend further until all the ingredients are mixed in thoroughly.

8. When the pumpkin is done, take the baking sheet out of the oven. Let it cool for a few minutes and then peel off the skins. Add the pumpkin pieces to the food processor with the cream and blend until thoroughly mixed.

9. Pour the mixture into a pot and simmer over medium heat. Add enough water or broth to thin out the soup according to your preference.

10. Garnish with pumpkin seeds and serve hot.

## Macros

- 30g fat

- 6.5g protein □ 18g carbs

- 500 calories

# DINNER

## INDONESIAN CHICKEN

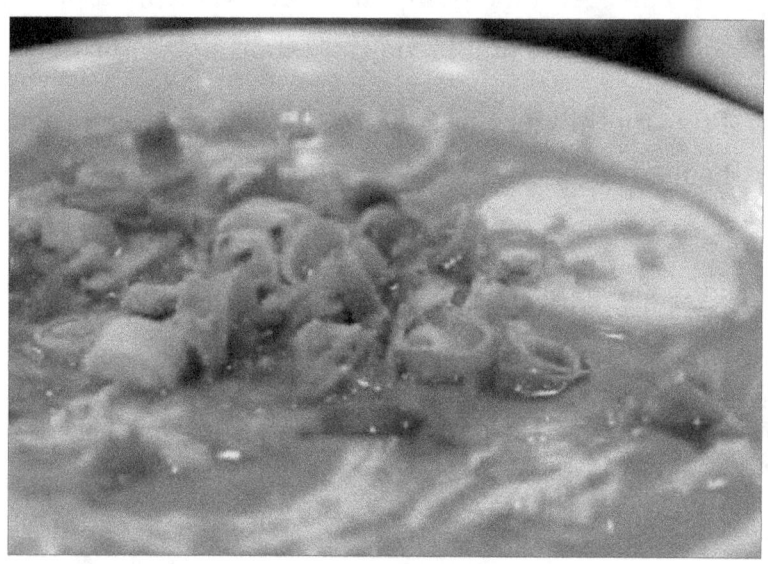

Servings: 4

### Ingredients

- 2 tablespoon olive oil

- pounds chicken thighs (deboned, skin removed)

- medium tomatoes, chopped

- 1 cup chicken broth

- 1 14-ounce can of coconut milk, unsweetened

- 1 tablespoon lime juice

- cup white onion, chopped

- cloves garlic, chopped

- 1 ounce of peanuts, toasted 3 small red chili, chopped

- 1 tablespoon ginger, grated

- tablespoon water

- teaspoons coriander, ground

- 1 teaspoon turmeric, ground

- 1 teaspoon cinnamon, ground

- 1 teaspoon cumin, ground

- 1 teaspoon fennel seed, ground

- 1/2 teaspoon black pepper

## Directions:

1. For the spice paste, combine all the ingredients for the paste and blend in a food processor until the consistency is smooth.

2. For the Balinese chicken curry, cut the chicken into 2-inch cubes.

3. Heat a large pan and cook the spice paste in olive oil for about three to four minutes while stirring.

4. Add the chicken to the paste and cook for a further two minutes.

5. Stir the tomatoes and chicken stock into the chicken and paste mixture.

6. After the mixture has begun to simmer, turn the heat down to a minimum and cook for 30 minutes more.

7. Add the coconut milk and cook for 20 minutes more while stirring.

8. Add the lime juice and season with salt and pepper.

## Macros

- 22g fat
- 53g protein
- 7g carbs
- 430 calories

# TUESDAY BREAKFAST

## KETO COCONUT

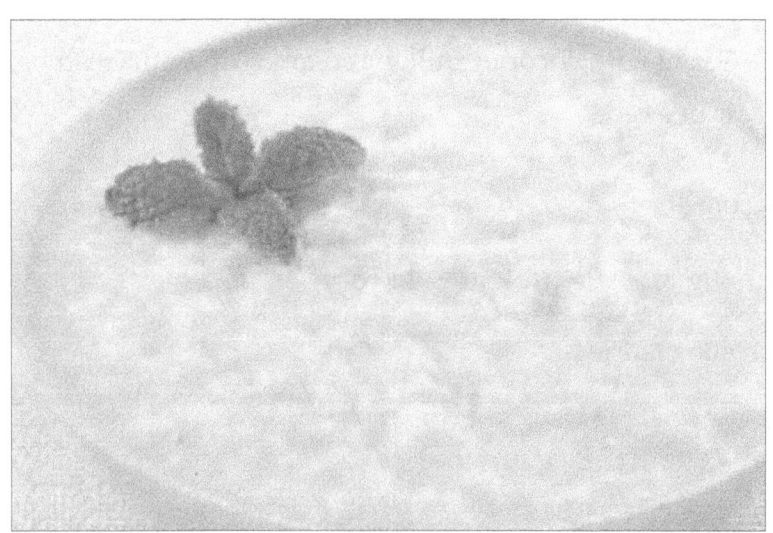

Servings: 1

## Ingredients

- 1 oz butter or coconut oil

- 1 egg

- 1 tbsp coconut flour

- 1 pinch ground psyllium husk powder

- 4 tbsp coconut cream

- 1 pinch salt

## Directions:

1. Add all ingredients to a non-stick saucepan. Mix well and put over low heat, stirring continuously until you achieve your desired texture.

2. Serve with coconut milk or cream. Top with fresh berries if desired.

## Macros

- 49g fat □ 9g protein □ 4g carbs
- 486 calories

# LUNCH

## HEARTY LAMB MEATBALLS WITH CAULIFLOWER RICE RECIPE

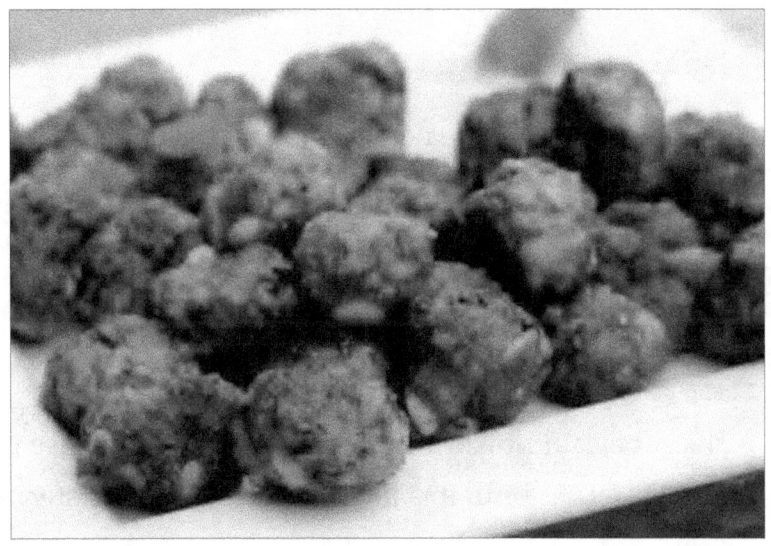

Servings: 5

## **Ingredients**

- 200 grams cauliflower

- Salt and pepper to taste

- 1 pound lamb, minced

- 1 large egg

- 1 teaspoon salt

- 1 teaspoon fennel seed

- 1 teaspoon garlic powder

- 1 teaspoon pepper

- 1 teaspoon paprika 2 tablespoons coconut oil

- ½ yellow onion, chopped

- 4 grams garlic, minced finely

- 1 bunch fresh mint leaves chopped roughly

- 1 tablespoon lemon zest

- 4 ounces cheese (goat milk cheese is recommended)

## Directions:

1. Place the cauliflower in a food processor and pulse it for a few minutes until it is the same size and consistency as rice.

2. Lightly oil a pan and cook the cauliflower rice for about 8 minutes while covered. Season it with salt and pepper.

3. Mix the lamb, egg, and spices in a bowl with your hands until thoroughly combined. Form the mixture into meatballs. You should be able to make around 12 to 15 meatballs.

4. Place a few meatballs on top of each portion and top with mint leaves, lemon zest, and goat cheese.

5. Place a skillet over medium heat and drizzle in the coconut oil. Cook the onion until it's translucent, which should take 5 to 8 minutes.

6. Add the garlic and cook for a few more minutes.

7. Add the meatballs to the pan and cook all sides evenly until they are firm.

8. Divide the cauliflower rice into four portions.

## Macros

- 41g fat
- 27g protein
- 3.5g carbs
- 495 calories

# DINNER

## SPICY STEAK

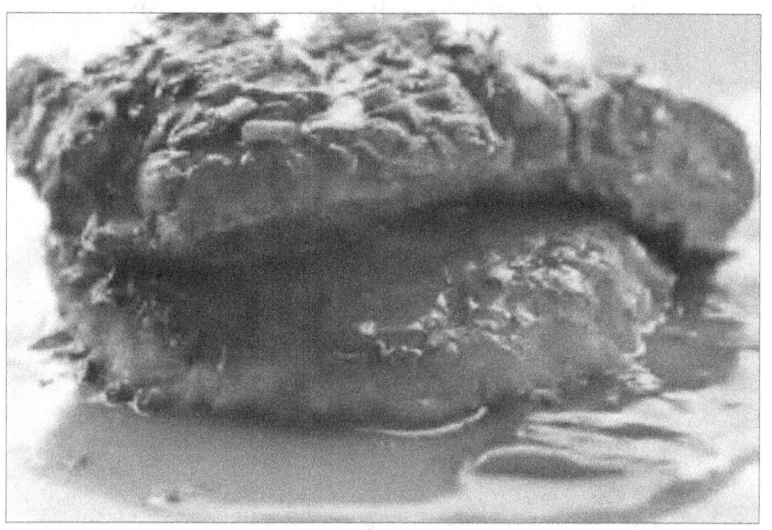

Servings: 2

## <u>Ingredients</u>

- 16 ounces skirt steak

- Salt and pepper to taste

- 1 cup guacamole

- 4 ounces cheese (pepper jack is recommended)

- 1 cup sour cream

- 1 handful cilantro

- A few drops of Tabasco sauce

## Directions:

1. Season the meat with salt and pepper.

2. Place a cast iron skillet on the stove over high heat.

3. When the pan is hot enough, cook the meat for 3 to 4 minutes on each side.

4. Remove the meat from the heat and let it rest to bring out the juices.

5. After a few minutes, slice the steak into thin strips. You should have enough for four servings.

6. Grate the cheese sprinkle over each serving of steak.

7. Top with guacamole and sour cream. You may also add a few drops of Tabasco sauce if you wish.

8. Garnish with cilantro.

## Macros

- 50g fat

- 33g protein

- 5.5g carbs

- 620 calories

# WEDNESDAY BREAKFAST

## KETO FRIED EGGS WITH KALE AND

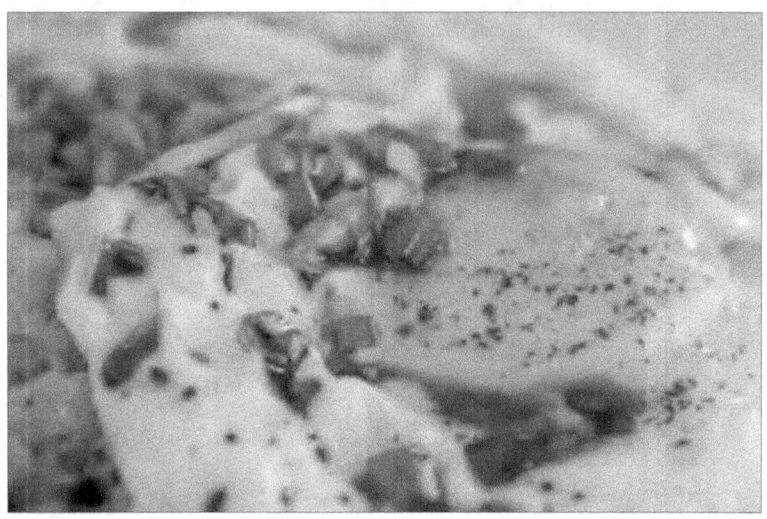

Servings: 2

## Ingredients

- ¼ lb kale

- 1 ½ oz butter

- 3 oz smoked pork belly or bacon

- 2 tbsp frozen cranberries

- ½ oz pecans or walnuts

- 2 eggs

- Salt and pepper

## Directions:

1 . Trim and chop kale into large squares. Melt 2/3 of the butter in a frying pan and fry kale quickly on high heat until slightly brown around the edges.

2 . Remove kale from pan and set aside. Sear the meat in the same pan until crispy.

3 . Lower heat, return sautéed kale to the pan and add cranberries and nuts. Stir until thoroughly warmed. Put aside in a bowl.

4 . Turn the heat back up to fry the eggs using the remaining butter, salt, and pepper to taste.

5 . Plate the eggs with the greens and serve immediately

## Macros

- 99g fat

- 26g protein

- 8g carbs

- 1033 calories

# LUNCH

## CAULIFLOWER SOUP WITH

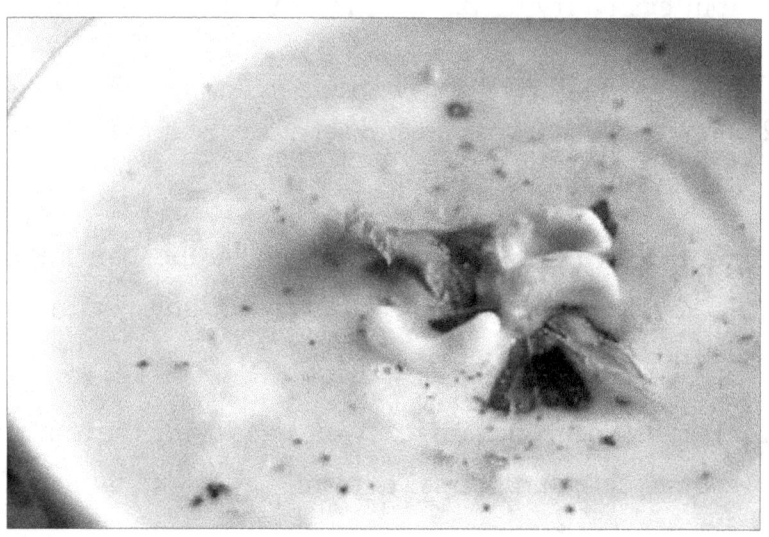

Servings: 4

### **Ingredients**

- 4 cups of chicken or vegetable stock, and 1 lb of cauliflower

- 7 ounces of cream cheese

- 4 ounces of butter

- 7-8 ounces of diced pancetta or bacon

- 3 ounces of nuts (pecan)

- 1 tablespoon of butter, Dijon mustard, and paprika powder Salt and pepper to taste

## Directions:

1. Cut the vegetables and cauliflower into smaller pieces (smaller florets) because it will help cook the soup faster.

2. Grab a good chunk of cauliflower and cut into quarter-inch pieces

3. Sauté the pancetta and cauliflower in butter until they both get crispy.

4. Towards the end, add some paprika and nuts to enhance flavor.

5. Boil the cauliflower florets until they get softer. Put butter, cream cheese and mustard in the mix.

6. Blend it until it gets to your desired consistency then add some salt and pepper.

7. The soup gets creamier the longer you blend it.

8. Serve the meal in bowls then add the pancetta and cauliflower crumbles on top.

## Macros

- 37g fat

- 13g protein
- 10g carbs
- 240 calories

# DINNER

## OLD FASHIONED SHEPHERD'S PIE

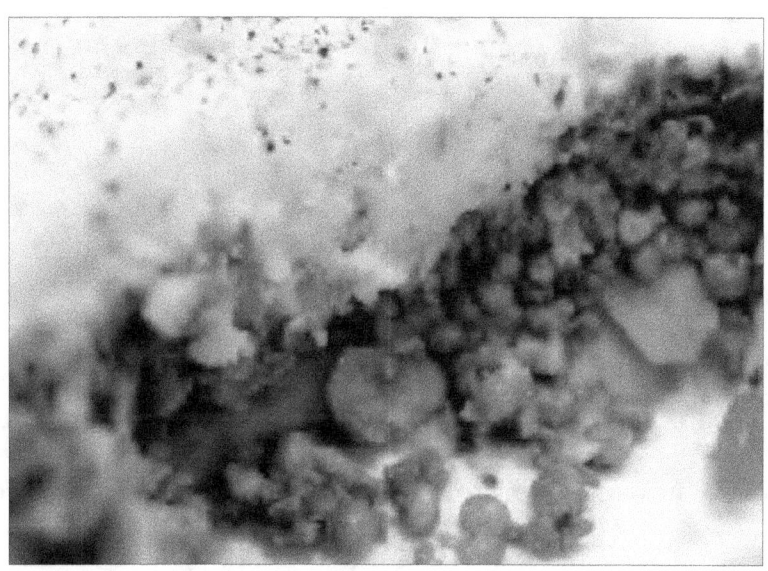

Servings: 4

### Ingredients

- 1/4 cup coconut oil

- 1 pound turkey, lamb or beef, minced

- 1/4 cup yellow onion, finely chopped

- 3 cloves garlic, minced

- 1/2 cup celery, chopped

- cup tomatoes, diced

- 12 ounces of riced cauliflower (cook and drained beforehand)

- 1 cup heavy cream

- 1 cup cheese, shredded

- 1/4 cup parmesan, grated

- 1 teaspoon thyme

## Directions:

1. Heat 1/4 cup of oil in a skillet.

2. Sauté the ground meat, onions, garlic, and celery in the pan. You'll know it is ready when the meat is brown.

3. Remove the pan from the heat and mix in the tomatoes. Transfer everything to a casserole dish.

4. Blend the cauliflower, cream, thyme, and the cheese in a good processor. Aim for a consistency similar to that of mashed potatoes

5. Spread the cauliflower mixture over the meat.

6. Place the casserole dish in the oven and bake for 35 to 40 minutes at 350°F.

7. When done, let the dish cool slightly before cutting into portions

## Macros

- 39g fat

- 23g protein

- 6g carbs

- 469 calories

# THURSDAY BEAKFAST

## KETO MUSHROOM OMELET RECIPE

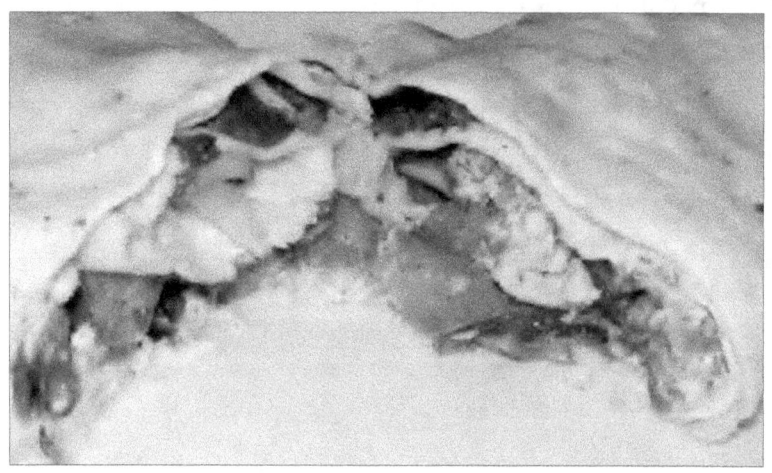

Servings : 1

## Ingredients

- 3 eggs

- 1 oz butter

- 1 oz shredded cheese

- 1/5 yellow onion

- 3 mushrooms

- Salt and pepper

## Directions:

1. Crack eggs into a mixing bowl with a pinch of salt and pepper. Whisk together eggs with a fork until smooth and frothy.

2. Add seasoning to taste.

3. Melt butter in a frying pan, then pour in the egg mixture.

4. When omelet begins to become firm but retains some raw egg on top, sprinkle cheese, mushrooms, and onion on top (optional).

5. Using a spatula, carefully ease around the edges of the omelet to fold it over in half.

6. Once the omelet is golden brown underneath, remove the pan from the heat and slide the omelet onto a plate.

## Macros

- 43g fat
- 25g protein
- 4g carbs
- 510 calories

# LUNCH

## KETO BLT WITH CLOUD

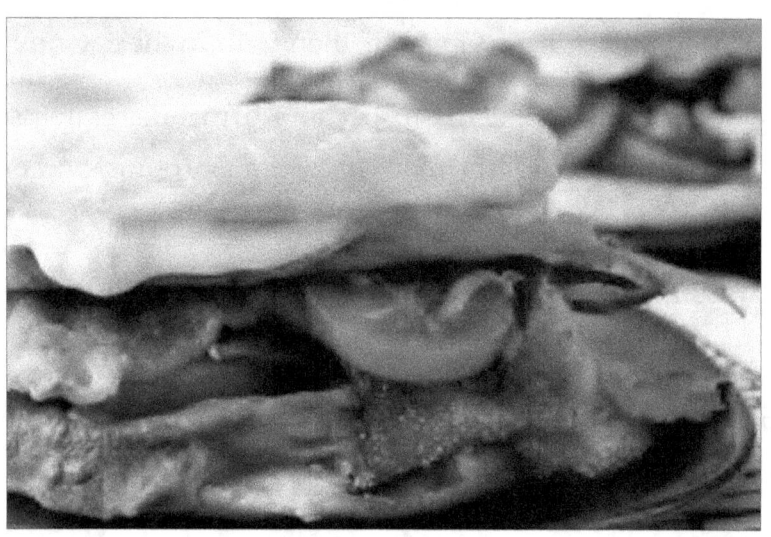

Servings: 4

### Ingredients

- Cloud bread 3 eggs

- 4¼ oz. cream cheese

- 1 pinch salt

- ½ tbsp ground psyllium husk powder

- ½ tsp baking powder

- ¼ tsp cream of tartar (optional)

- Toppings

- 8 tbsp mayonnaise

- 5 oz. bacon

- 2 oz. lettuce 1 tomato, thinly sliced fresh basil (optional)

## Directions:

1. Preheat oven to 300°F (150°C).

2. Separate the eggs. Put the egg whites in one bowl and the yolks in another.

3. Whip egg whites together with salt (and cream of tartar, if you are using any) until very stiff.

4. Preferably using a handheld electric mixer, you should be able to turn the bowl over without the egg whites moving.

5. Add cream cheese to the egg yolks and mix well. To make it more bread-like, add in the optional psyllium seed husk and baking powder.

6. Gently fold the egg whites into the egg yolk mixture. Try to keep the air in the egg whites.

7. Put 8 cloud bread pieces on a paper-lined baking tray.

8. Bake in the middle of the oven for about 25 minutes, until they turn golden.

9. Start building the BLT,

10. Fry the bacon in a skillet on medium-high heat until crispy.

11. Place the cloud bread pieces top-side down.

12. Spread 1–2 tablespoons of mayonnaise on each.

13. Place lettuce, tomato, some finely chopped fresh basil and fried bacon in layers between the bread halves.

14. Serve immediately.

## Macros

- 48g fat

- 11g protein

- 4g carbs

- 498 calories

# DINNER

## KETO PESTO CHICKEN CASSEROLE WITH FETA CHEESE AND OLIVES RECIPE

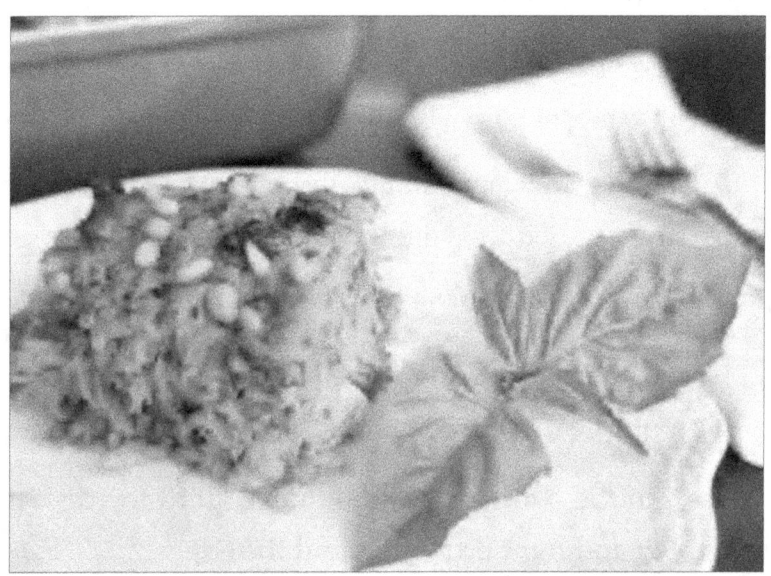

Servings: 4

### Ingredients

- 25 oz. boneless chicken thighs or chicken breasts

- 1 oz. butter, for frying

- 3 oz. red pesto or green pesto

- 1¼ cups heavy whipping cream

- 3 oz. pitted olives

- 5 oz. feta cheese, diced 1 garlic clove, finely chopped salt, and pepper 5 oz. leafy greens 4 tbsp olive oil sea salt and ground black pepper

## Directions:

1. Preheat the oven to 400°F (200°C).

2. Cut the chicken thighs or chicken breasts into bite-sized pieces. Season with salt and pepper.

3. Add butter to a large skillet and fry the chicken pieces in batches on medium-high heat until golden brown.

4. Mix pesto and heavy cream in a bowl.

5. Place the fried chicken pieces in a baking dish together with olives, feta cheese, and garlic. Add the pesto.

6. Bake in the oven for 20-30 minutes, until the dish turns bubbly and light brown around the edges.

## Macros

- 96g fat

- 39g protein

- 6g carbs

- 1044 calories

# FRIDAY BREAKFAST

## MARIA'S KETO PANCAKES

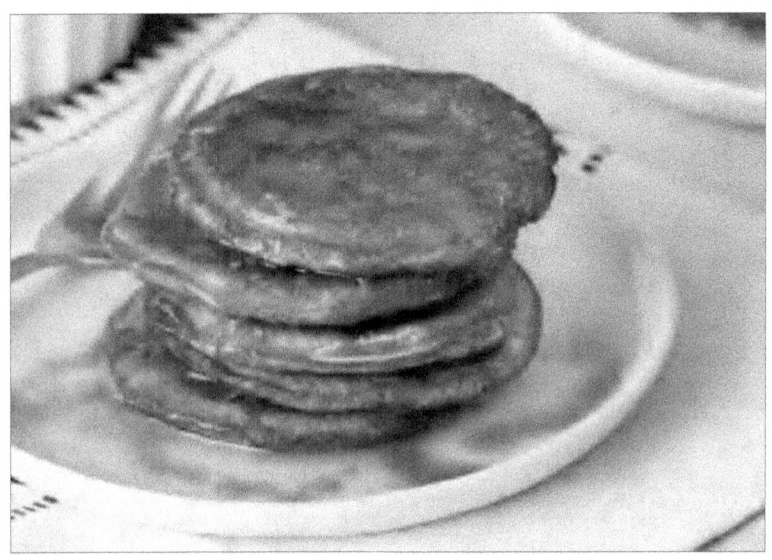

Servings: 1

### Ingredients

- 2/3 oz pork rinds

- 2 eggs

- 2 tbsp unsweetened cashew milk

- 1 tsp maple extract

- tsp ground cinnamon

- tbsp coconut oil for frying

## Directions:

1. Place pork rinds in a blender and pulse until finely ground into a powder. Add the rest of the ingredients and combine until smooth.

2. Heat a skillet to medium heat. Once hot, add a tablespoon of coconut oil.

3. Pour ¼ cup batter into the skillet. Fry until golden brown and set, which will take about 2 minutes. Flip and continue to cook until cooked all the way through.

4. Remove from skillet and repeat with remaining batter. Add more coconut oil as needed.

## Macros

- 43g fat
- 24g protein
- 2g carbs
- 510 calories

# LUNCH

## FATHEAD PIZZA

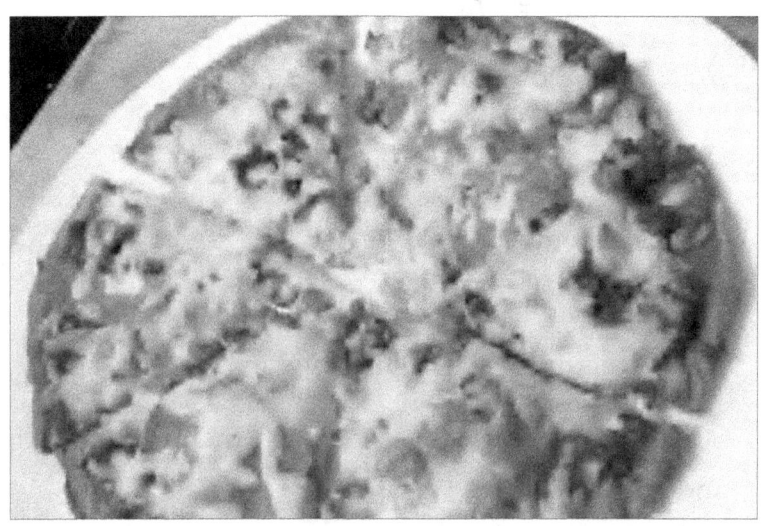

Servings: 2

## Ingredients

- Crust

- 1½ cups shredded mozzarella cheese

- ¾ cup almond flour

- 2 tbsp cream cheese

- 1 tsp white wine vinegar

- 1 egg ½ tsp salt olive oil to grease your hands Toppings

- 8 oz. fresh Italian sausage

- 1 tbsp butter

- ½ cup unsweetened tomato sauce

- ½ tsp dried oregano

- 1½ cups shredded mozzarella cheese

## Directions:

1. Preheat the oven to 400°F (200°C).

2. Heat mozzarella and cream cheese in a small, non-stick pan on medium heat or in a bowl in the microwave oven.

3. Stir until they melt together. Add the other ingredients and mix well.

4. Moisten your hands with olive oil and flatten the dough on parchment paper, making a circle about 8 inches (20 cm) in diameter. You can also use a rolling pin to flatten the dough between two sheets of parchment paper.

5. Remove the top parchment sheet (if used). Prick the crust with a fork (all over) and bake in the oven for 10–12 minutes until golden brown. Remove from the oven.

6. While the crust is baking, sautée the ground sausage meat in olive oil or butter.

7 . Spread a thin layer of tomato sauce on the crust. Top the pizza with meat and plenty of cheese. Bake for 10–15 minutes or until the cheese has melted.

8 . Sprinkle oregano on top and serve with a green salad.

## Macros

- 110g fat
- 67g protein
- 10g carbs
- 1316 calories

# DINNER

## KETO MEAT PIE

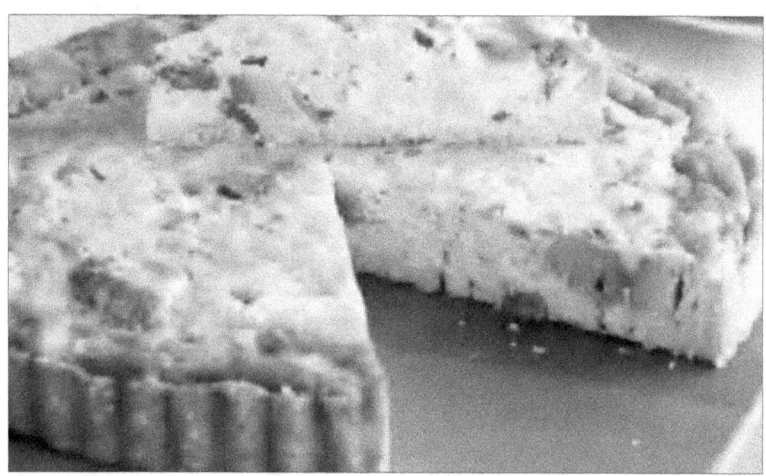

Servings : 6

### Ingredients

- The filling

- ½ yellow onion, finely chopped

- garlic clove, finely chopped

- tbsp butter or olive oil 20 oz. ground beef or ground lamb salt and pepper 1 tbsp dried oregano or dried basil

- 4 tbsp tomato paste or ajvar relish

- ½ cup of water

- Pie crust ¾ cup almond flour

- 4 tbsp sesame seeds

- 4 tbsp coconut flour

- 1 tbsp ground psyllium husk powder

- 1 tsp baking powder

- 1 pinch salt

- 3 tbsp olive oil or coconut oil

- 1 egg

- 4 tbsp water

- Topping

- 8 oz. cottage cheese

- 7 oz. shredded cheese

## Directions:

1. Preheat the oven to 350°F (175°C).

2. Fry onion and garlic in butter or olive oil over medium heat for a few minutes, until the onion is soft. Add the ground beef and keep frying. Add oregano or basil and add salt and pepper to taste.

3. Add tomato paste, pesto or ajvar relish – use what you have on hand. Add water. Lower the heat and let simmer

for at least 20 minutes. While the meat simmers, make the dough for the crust.

4. Mix all the dough ingredients in a food processor for a few minutes until the dough turns into a ball. If you don't have a food processor, you can mix by hand with a fork.

5. Place a round piece of parchment paper in a well-greased springform pan — 9-10 inches in diameter — to make it easier to remove the pie when it's done. (You can also use a deep-dish pie pan.) Spread the dough in the pan and up along the sides. Use a spatula or well-greased fingers.

6. Pre-bake the crust for 10-15 minutes. Take it out of the oven and place the meat in the crust. Mix cottage cheese and shredded cheese together, and layer on top of the pie.

7. Bake for 30-40 minutes on a lower rack or until the pie has turned a golden color.

8. Serve with a fresh green salad and dressing.

## Macros

- 47g fat
- 38g protein
- 7g carbs
- 622 calories

# SATURDAY BREAKFAST

## KETO BISCUITS AND GRAVY

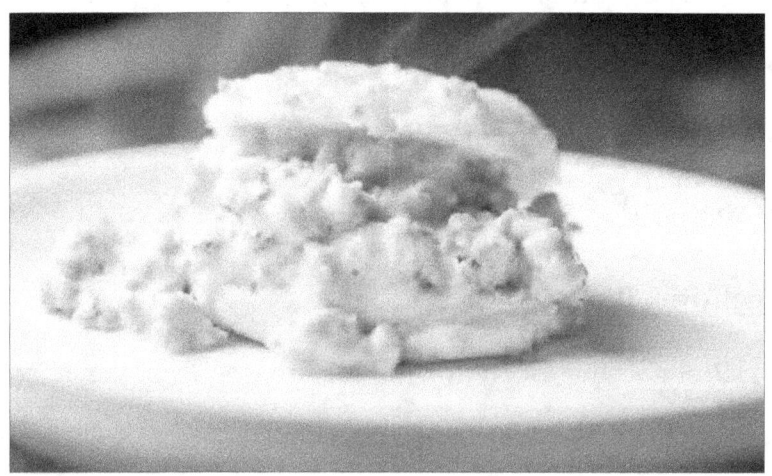

Servings: 4

## Ingredients:

- Biscuits

- ¼ cup almond flour

- 1/10 tsp sea salt

- ¼ tsp baking powder

- 1 egg white

- ½ tbsp very cold butter or coconut oil

- ¼ tsp garlic powder or seasoning of your preference (optional)

- ¼ tsp coconut oil cooking spray

## Ingredients: Gravy

- 2 ½ oz crumbled fresh sausage, preferably pork

- ¼ cup cream cheese or coconut cream

- ¼ cup beef broth or chicken broth

- Salt and pepper

## Directions: Biscuits

1. Preheat the oven to 400°F. Grease a cookie sheet or muffin pan with coconut oil spray.

2. Beat the egg whites until very fluffy and firm.

3. In a separate medium bowl, mix the baking powder into the almond flour.

4. Cut in cold butter and salt (the cold butter is what makes the biscuits flaky). Gently fold in the dry mixture into the egg whites.

5. Spoon a dollop of the dough onto the cookie sheet (or muffin tin) and bake for 11-15 minutes.

## Directions: Gravy

1. Cook sausage in a large skillet on medium heat for 5-6 minutes or until thoroughly heated, stirring frequently.

2. Gradually add cream cheese and broth. Cook until mixture comes to a soft simmer and thickens, stirring constantly until smooth.

3. Reduce heat to medium-low. Simmer about 2 minutes, stirring continuously. Season to taste with salt and pepper.

4. Split biscuits in half and place 2 halves on each plate. Serve with about 1/3 cup gravy.

## Macros

- 33g fat
- 13g protein
- 3g carbs
- 358 calories

# LUNCH

## KETO HAMBURGER PATTLES WITH CREAMY TOMATO SAUCE AND FRIED CABBAGE RECIPE

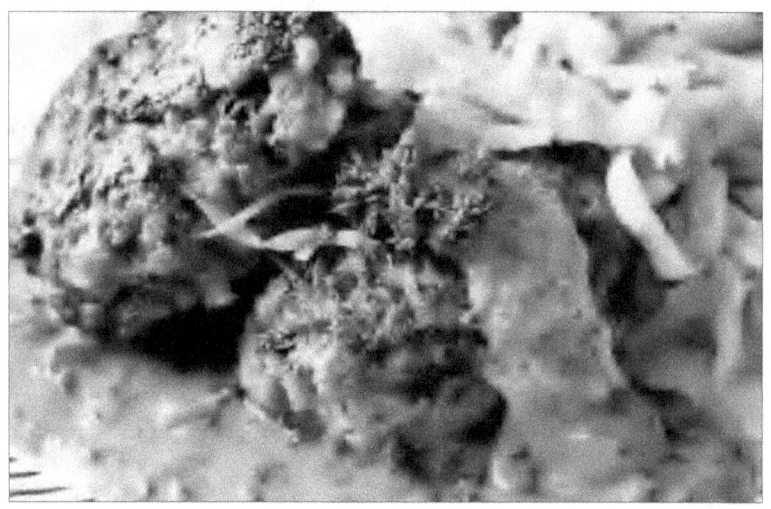

Servings: 4

### Ingredients

**Hamburger Patties**

- 25 oz. ground beef

- 1 egg

- 3 oz. crumbled feta cheese 1 tsp salt

172

- ¼ tsp ground black pepper

- 2 oz. fresh parsley, finely chopped

- 1 tbsp olive oil, for frying

- 1 oz. butter, for frying

## Gravy

- ¾ cup heavy whipping cream

- oz. fresh parsley, coarsely chopped

- tbsp tomato paste or ajvar relish

- Salt and pepper

- Fried green cabbage

- 25 oz. shredded green cabbage

- 4¼ oz. butter

- Salt and pepper

## Directions:

1. Add all ingredients for the hamburgers to a large bowl. Blend it using a wooden spoon or your clean hands. Don't over mix since that can make your patties tough. Use wet hands to form eight oblong patties.

2. Add butter and olive oil to a large frying pan. Fry over medium-high heat for at least 10 minutes or until the

patties have turned a nice color. Flip them a few times for even cooking.

3. Add tomato paste and whipping cream to the pan when the patties are almost done. Stir and let simmer for a few minutes. Add salt and pepper to taste.

4. Sprinkle chopped parsley on top before serving.

5. Start butter-frying the green cabbage.

6. Shred the cabbage finely using a food processor or sharp knife.

7. Add butter to a large frying pan.

8. Place the pan over medium high heat and sauté the shredded cabbage for at least 15 minutes or until the cabbage is wilted and golden brown around the edges.

9. Stir regularly and lower the heat a little towards the end. Add salt and pepper to taste.

## Macros

- 78g fat
- 43g protein
- 10g carbs
- 924 calories

# DINNER

## KETO LASAGNA

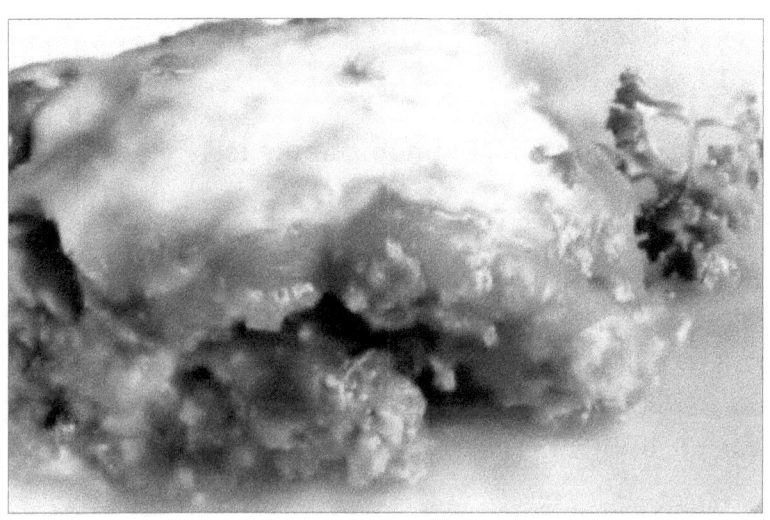

Servings: 6

### Ingredients

- 2 tbsp olive oil 1 yellow onion

- 1 garlic clove

- 20 oz. ground beef

- 3 tbsp tomato paste

- ½ tbsp dried basil

- 1 tsp salt

- ¼ tsp ground black pepper

- ½ cup of water

- Keto pasta 8 eggs

- 10 oz. cream cheese

- 1 tsp salt

- 5 tbsp ground psyllium husk powder

- Cheese topping

- 2 cups crème fraîche or sour cream

- 5 oz. shredded cheese

- 2 oz. grated parmesan cheese

- ½ tsp salt

- ¼ tsp ground black pepper

- ½ cup fresh parsley, finely chopped

## Directions:

1. Start with the ground beef mixture, perhaps even the day before, for a more flavorful result.

2. Peel and finely chop onion and garlic and fry in olive oil until soft. Add the ground beef and fry until golden. Add tomato paste and spices.

3. Stir thoroughly and add water. Bring to a boil, lower the heat, and let simmer for at least 15 minutes or until most of the water has evaporated. Since the lasagna sheets used here don't soak up as much liquid as regular ones, the mixture should be quite dry.

4. Meanwhile, make the lasagna sheets according to the instructions below.

5. Preheat the oven to 400°F (200°C). Mix shredded cheese with sour cream and most of the Parmesan cheese. Reserve one or two tablespoons for topping. Add salt and pepper and stir in the parsley.

6. Place lasagna sheets and pasta sauce in layers in a greased 9" x 13" baking dish.

7. Spread the crème fraîche mixture and the remaining Parmesan cheese on top.

8. Bake in the oven for about 30 minutes or until the lasagna has a nicely browned surface.

9. Serve with a green salad and your favorite dressing.

10. Start making the lasagna sheets.

11. Preheat the oven to 300°F (150°C). Add eggs, cream cheese and salt to a medium-sized bowl and mix into a smooth batter. Continue to whisk while adding in the ground psyllium husk powder, a little at a time. Let sit for a few minutes.

12. Spread the batter on a baking sheet lined with parchment paper using a spatula. Place another parchment paper on top and flatten with a rolling pin until the batter is at least 13" x 18" (33 x 45 cm). You can also divide into two batches and use another baking sheet for an even thinner pasta.

13. Let both pieces of parchment paper remain in place. Bake for about 10-12 minutes. Let cool and remove the paper, slice into sheets that fit your baking dish.

## Macros

- 76g fat

- 42g protein

- 9g carbs

- 901 calories

# SUNDAY BREAKFAST

## KETO MUSHROOM AND CHEESE FRITTATA RECIPE

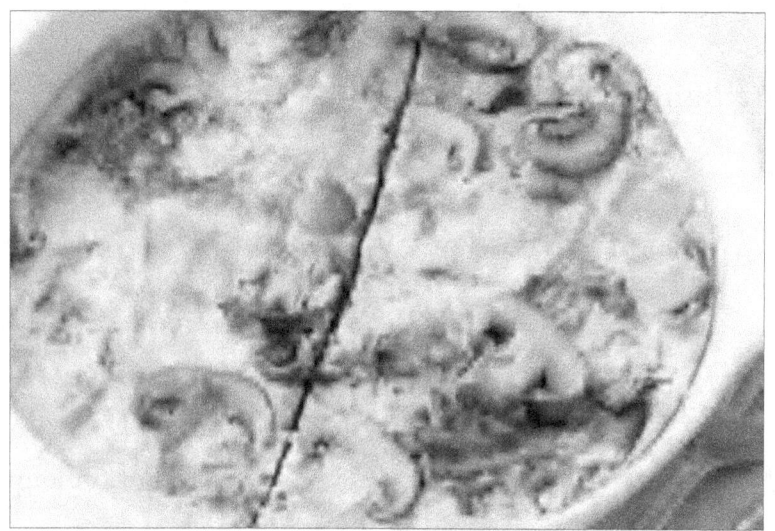

Servings: 4

### Ingredients:

- Frittata 15 oz mushrooms

- 3 oz butter

- 6 scallions

- 1/2 tsp ground black pepper

- 10 eggs

- 1 tsp salt

- 1 tbsp fresh parsley

- 8 oz shredded cheese

- 1 cup mayonnaise

- 4 oz leafy greens

## Ingredients: Vinaigrette

- 4 tbsp olive oil

- 1 tbsp white wine vinegar ½ tsp salt

- ¼ tsp ground black pepper

## Directions:

1. Preheat oven to 350ºF. First, mix together vinaigrette ingredients and set aside.

2. Slice the mushrooms to your preference.

3. Sauté mushrooms over medium-high heat with most of the butter until golden, then lower the heat. Save the remaining butter to grease the baking dish.

4. Chop scallions and mix into the fried mushrooms. Add salt and pepper to taste and mix in parsley.

5. Mix eggs, mayonnaise, and cheese in a separate bowl. Add salt and pepper to taste.

6. Add the mushrooms and scallions and pour everything into a well-greased baking dish.

7. Bake for 30-40 minutes or until the frittata turns golden and the eggs are cooked.

8. Let cool for 5 minutes and serve with leafy greens and the vinaigrette.

## Macros

- 101g fat
- 32g protein
- 6g carbs
- 1061 calories

# LUNCH

## KETO

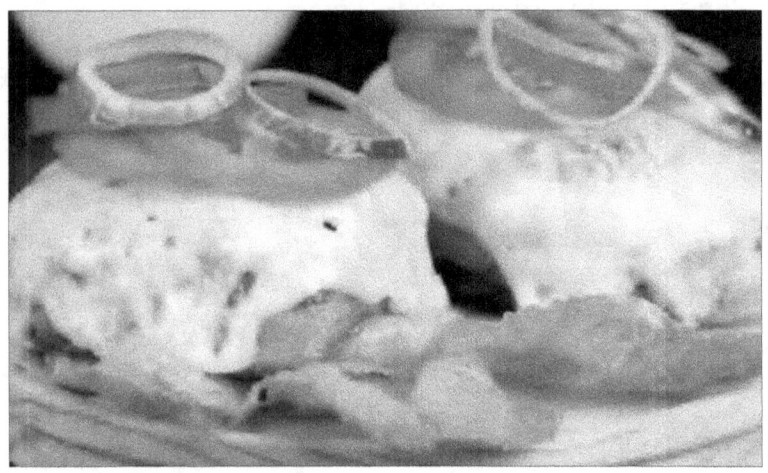

Servings:4

## **Ingredients**

- 25 oz. ground beef

- 7 oz. shredded cheese 2 tsp garlic powder

- 2 tsp onion powder

- 2 tsp paprika powder

- 2 tbsp fresh oregano, finely chopped

- 2 oz. butter, for frying

- Salsa

- 2 tomatoes

- 2 scallions

- 1 avocado

- 1 tbsp olive oil salt fresh cilantro, to taste Toppings

- ¾ cup mayonnaise

- 5 oz. cooked bacon 4 tbsp Dijon mustard

- ½ cup sliced dill pickles

- 5 oz. lettuce

- ¼ cup pickled jalapeños

## Directions:

1. Chop up the salsa ingredients and stir together in a small bowl. Set aside.

2. Mix in seasoning and half the cheese into the ground beef.

3. Make four burgers and fry in a pan or grill if you prefer. Add the remaining cheese on top towards the end.

4. Serve on lettuce with dill pickle and mustard. And don't forget the homemade salsa!

## Macros

- 104g fat

- 54g protein

- 8g carbs

- 1204 calories

# DINNER

## KETO PULLED PORK

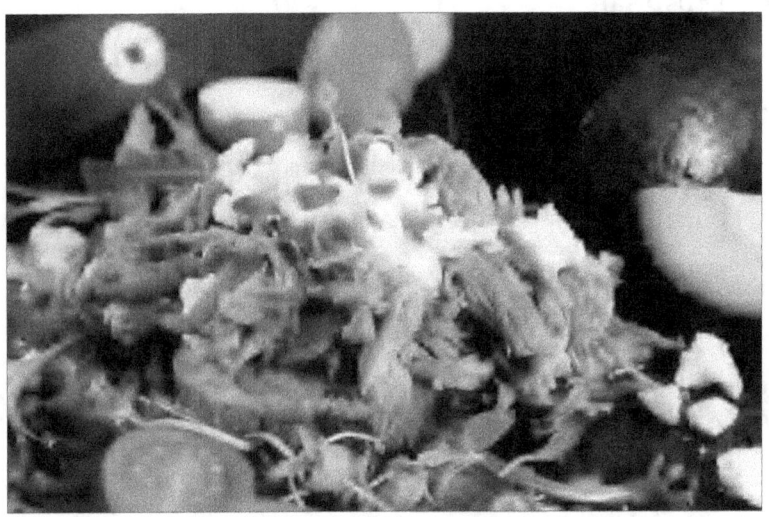

Servings: 4

### Ingredients

- 2 red onions

- whole garlic

- ¾ cup red wine

- ½ cup olive oil

- tbsp coriander seed, crushed

- 2 tsp dried thyme

- 2 tsp ground black pepper

- tsp ground cinnamon

- lbs pork shoulder

- 1 tbsp salt

## Directions:

1. Peel and slice the red onions into thin wedges. Cut the garlic cloves in half. Mix all the ingredients for the marinade. Place a large freezer bag inside a larger freezer bag, and add half the onion mix to the bag.

2. Rinse the pork collar, dry it well, and rub it all over with salt. Place the collar in the freezer bag and pour the marinade over it. Press out all air from the bag, seal the bag shut, and place it in a bowl. Leave the bowl in the refrigerator for at least 12 hours, preferably longer.

3. Preheat the oven to 260°F (125°C).

4. Place the meat, the rest of the onion mix and the marinade in an oven-safe casserole dish. Close it with a tight-fitting lid, and place the dish in the lower part of the oven for about 5 to 6 hours.

5. In the picture, the meat was cooked in an electric slow-cooker; it turned out extremely juicy and delicious. If using a slow-cooker, the meat will be ready in about 8 to

12 hours if set on low, but it also depends on the brand of the slow-cooker you're using.

6. To serve, pull the meat apart with two forks and mix it thoroughly with the gravy. Taste and adjust for salt. Serve this dish with low-carb bread, garlic butter, and coleslaw.

## Macros

- 89g fat
- 60g protein
- 11g carbs
- 1135 calories

# WEEK TWO
# MONDAY BREAKFAST
## CHEESY BACON AND

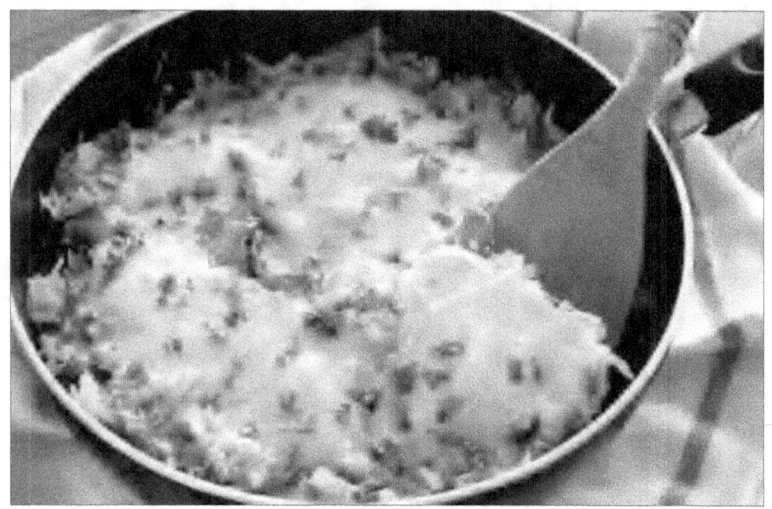

Servings: 4

## <u>Ingredients</u>

- 12 large eggs

- ½ cup spinach

- 12 pieces of bacon

- 1/3 cup cheese (ex. sharp cheddar) Salt and pepper to taste

## Directions:

1. Preheat oven to 400°F.

2. Fry bacon in a pan and set aside to drain.

3. Grease muffin pan with coconut or olive oil.

4. Line cups with one strip of bacon.

5. Beat eggs lightly.

6. Wrap spinach in a clean cloth or paper towel and wring out excess water.

7. Fold the spinach into the eggs.

8. Put the ¼ cup of this mixture into each cup of the muffin tray until ¾ full.

9. Sprinkle on cheese and season with salt and pepper.

10. Bake in the oven for 15 minutes or until done.

## Macros

- 7g fat

- 8g protein

- 1g carb

- 101 calories

# LUNCH
# KETO TORTILLA WITH GROUND BEEF AND SALSA RECIPE
## INGREDIENTS GROUND BEEF

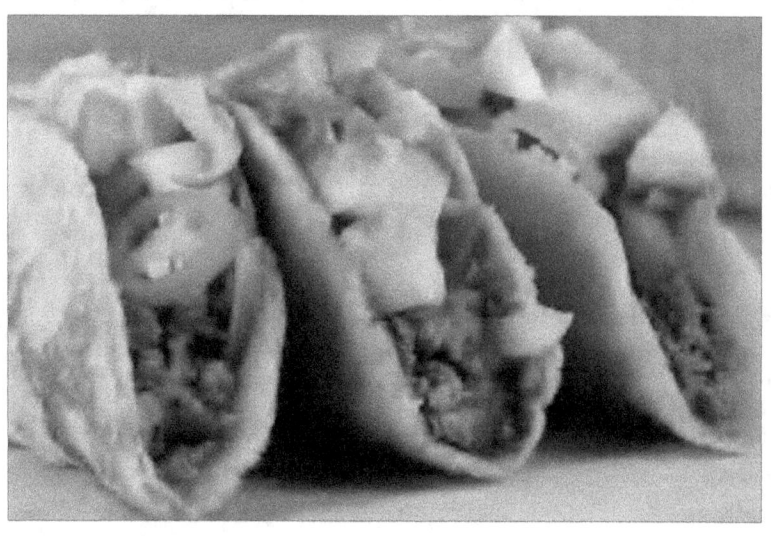

Servings: 4

- lb ground beef or ground lamb

- tbsp olive oil

- 2 tbsp Tex-Mex seasoning 1 cup of water salt and pepper Salsa

- 2 avocados

- 1 tomato, diced

- ½ cup fresh cilantro, chopped

- t bsp olive oil 1 lime, the juice salt and pepper Low-carb tortillas 2 eggs

- egg whites

- 5 oz. cream cheese

- 1½ tsp ground psyllium husk powder

- 1 tbsp coconut flour

- ½ tsp salt

- 1½ cups shredded Mexican cheese

- 3 oz. shredded lettuce

## Directions:

1. Low-carb tortillas

2. Preheat the oven to 400°F (200°C).

3. Whisk the eggs and egg whites fluffy and continue to whisk with a hand mixer, preferably for a few minutes. Add cream cheese and continue to whisk until the batter is smooth.

4. Mix salt, psyllium husk and coconut flour in a small bowl. Add the flour mix one spoon at a time into the

batter and continue to whisk some more. Let the batter sit for a few minutes, or until the batter is thick like an American pancake batter. How fast the batter will swell depends on the brand of psyllium husk – some trial and error might be needed.

5. Bring out two baking sheets and place parchment paper on each. Using a spatula, spread the batter thinly (no more than ¼ inch thick) into 4–6 circles or 2 rectangles.

6. Bake on the upper rack for about 5 minutes or more, until the tortilla turns a little brown around the edges. Carefully check the bottom side so that it doesn't burn.

7. **Filling 1**. Bring the ground beef out of the refrigerator a while before frying. Cold ground beef will cool down the frying pan and the ground beef will be boiled and not fried. That will make it taste a lot better.

8. Place a large frying pan over medium-high heat and heat up some oil. Add the ground beef and fry until cooked through.

9. Add the tex-mex seasoning and water and stir. Let simmer until most of the water is gone. Taste to see if it needs additional seasoning.

10. In the meantime, make the salsa from diced avocado, diced tomatoes, freshly squeezed lime juice, olive oil and a couple of handfuls of fresh cilantro. Add salt and pepper to taste.

11. Serve in a slice of tortilla bread, with shredded cheese and shredded leafy greens.

## Macros

- 66g fat
- 42g protein
- 9g carbs
- 821 calories

# DINNER

## KETO SALMON PIE

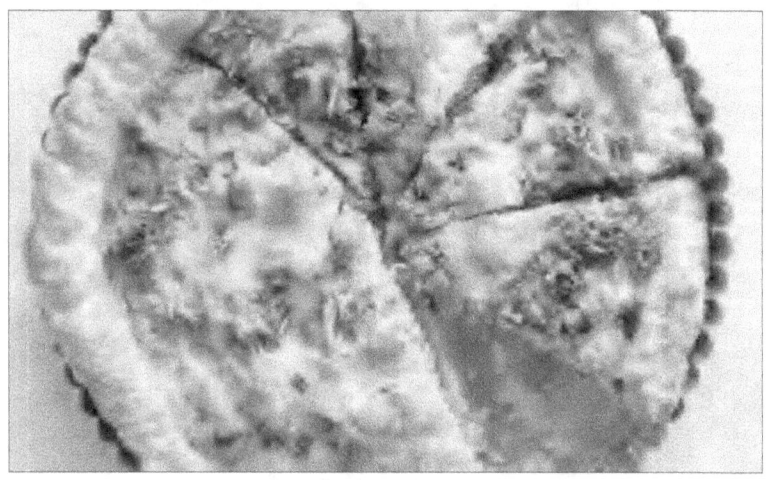

Servings : 4

## Ingredients

- Pie crust

- ¾ cup almond flour

- 4 tbsp sesame seeds

- 4 tbsp coconut flour

- 1 tbsp ground psyllium husk powder

- 1 tsp baking powder

- 1 pinch salt

- 3 tbsp olive oil or coconut oil

- 1 egg

- 4 tbsp water

- Filling

- 8 oz. smoked salmon

- 1 cup mayonnaise

- 3 eggs

- 2 tbsp fresh dill, finely chopped

- ½ tsp onion powder

- ¼ tsp ground black pepper

- 4¼ oz. cream cheese

- 1¼ cups shredded cheese

## Directions:

1. Preheat the oven to 350°F (175°C).

2. Place the pie dough ingredients into a food processor fitted with a plastic pastry blade. Pulse until mixture forms a ball. If you don't have a food processor, you can use a fork to mix the dough.

3. Fit a piece of parchment paper into a 10-inch (23-cm) springform pan. (This makes it a cinch to remove once it's cooked.)

4. Oil your fingers or a spatula, and gently press the dough into the springform pan. Prebake the crust for 10–15 minutes, or until lightly browned.

5. Mix all the ingredients for the filling, except the salmon, and pour that in the pie crust.

6. Add the salmon and bake for 35 minutes or until the pie is golden brown.

7. Let cool for a few minutes and serve with a salad or other vegetables.

## Macros

- 101g fat
- 58g protein
- 6g carbs
- 1179 calories

# TUESDAY BREAKFAST

## KETO CHEESE

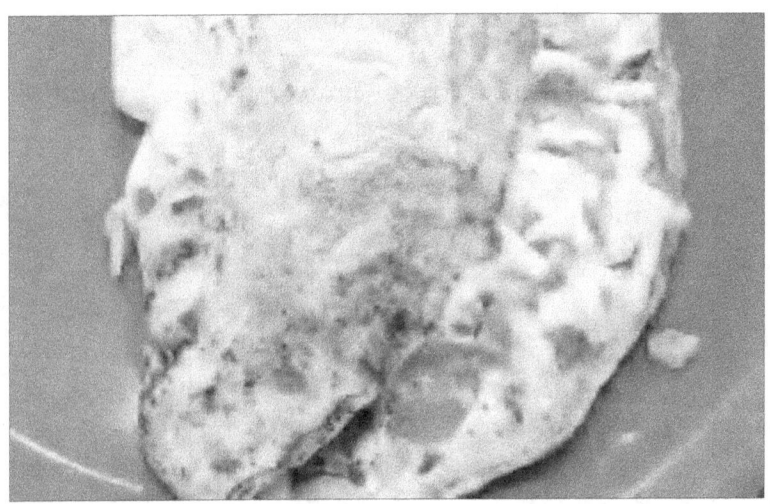

Servings: 2

## Ingredients

- 3 oz butter

- eggs

- oz shredded cheddar cheese Salt and pepper to taste

## Directions:

1. Whisk together eggs until smooth and slightly frothy. Blend half of the shredded cheddar into the mix, then add salt and pepper to taste.

2. Melt the butter in a hot frying pan. Add in the egg mixture and allow a few minutes to set.

3. Lower the heat and continue to cook until the egg mixture is almost fully cooked.

4. Add the remaining cheese, then fold and serve immediately.

## Macros

- 80g fat
- 40g protein
- 4g carbs
- 897 calories

# LUNCH

## KETO CHICKEN

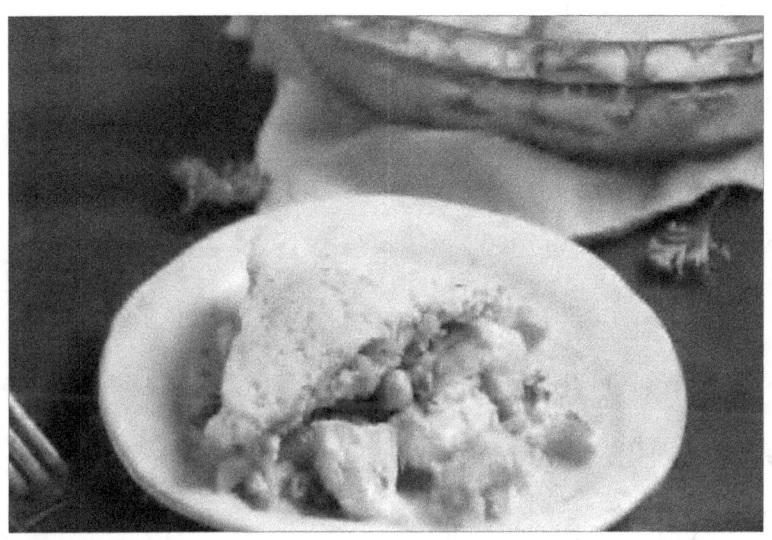

Servings:4

## Ingredients

### Pie crust

- ¾ cup almond flour

- 4 tbsp sesame seeds

- 4 tbsp coconut flour

- 1 tbsp ground psyllium husk powder

- 1 tsp baking powder

- 1 pinch salt

- 3 tbsp olive oil or coconut oil

- 1 egg

- 4 tbsp water

## Filling

- 10 oz. cooked chicken

- 1 cup mayonnaise

- 3 eggs

- ½ green bell pepper, finely chopped

- 1 tsp curry powder

- ½ tsp paprika powder

- ½ tsp onion powder

- ¼ tsp ground black pepper

- ½ cup cream cheese

- 1¼ cups shredded cheese

## Directions:

1. Preheat the oven to 350°F (175°C). Put all the ingredients for the pie crust into a food processor for a few minutes

until the dough firms up into a ball. If you don't have a food processor, you can also mix the dough with a fork.

2. Attach a piece of parchment paper to a springform pan, no larger than 10 inches (23 cm) in diameter (the springform pan makes it easier to remove the pie when it's done). Grease the bottom and sides of the pan.

3. Spread the dough into the pan. Use an oiled spatula or your fingers. Pre-bake the crust for 10–15 minutes.

4. Mix all other filling ingredients together, and fill the pie crust. Bake for 35–40 minutes or until the pie has turned a nice, golden brown.

5. Let cool and serve with salad and dressing.

## Macros

- 106g fat
- 37g protein
- 7g carbs
- 1146 calories

# DINNER

## GRILLED WHITE FISH WITH ZUCCINI AND KALE PESTO RECIPE

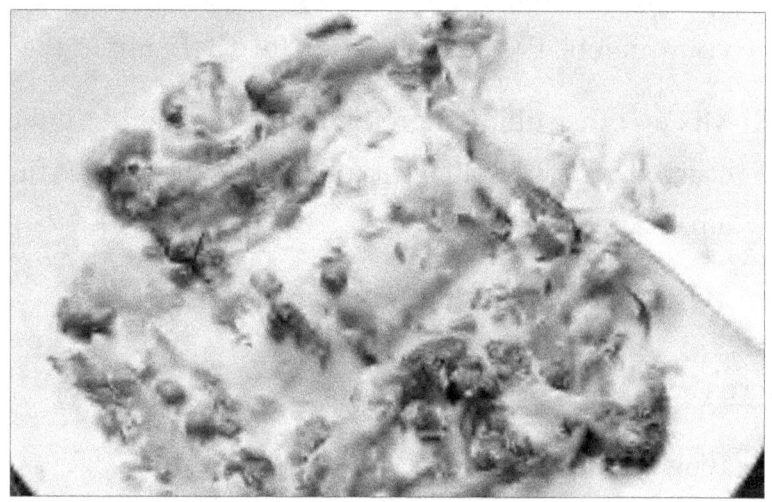

Servings: 4

### Ingredients

### Kale Pesto

- 3 oz. kale

- 3 tbsp lemon juice or lime juice

- 2 oz. walnuts

- garlic clove

- ½ tsp salt

- ¼ tsp ground black pepper

- ¾ cup olive oil

## Fish and zucchini

- zucchini

- tbsp lemon juice

- ½ tsp salt

- tbsp olive oil

- 1½ lbs white fish (thawed at room temperature, if frozen)

- ¼ tsp ground black pepper

## Directions:

1. Start preparing the pesto by chopping the kale roughly. Place the kale, walnuts, lime, and garlic in a blender or food processor, and purée until smooth. Season with salt and pepper. Add the oil towards the end and process a bit more. Set aside.

2. Rinse the zucchini and cut thinly with a sharp knife, slicer or mandolin. Put the slices in a bowl. Season with salt and pepper to taste, and dress with lemon juice and olive oil. Set aside.

3. Salt the fish on both sides and let sit for a few minutes. Wipe off excess liquid and brush with oil.

4. Grill or fry for a few minutes on each side. Add pepper and serve together with the zucchini and pesto.

## <u>Macros</u>

- 67g fat

- 38g protein

- 7g carbs

- 778 calories

# WEDNESDAY BREAKFAST

## KETO SEAFOOD

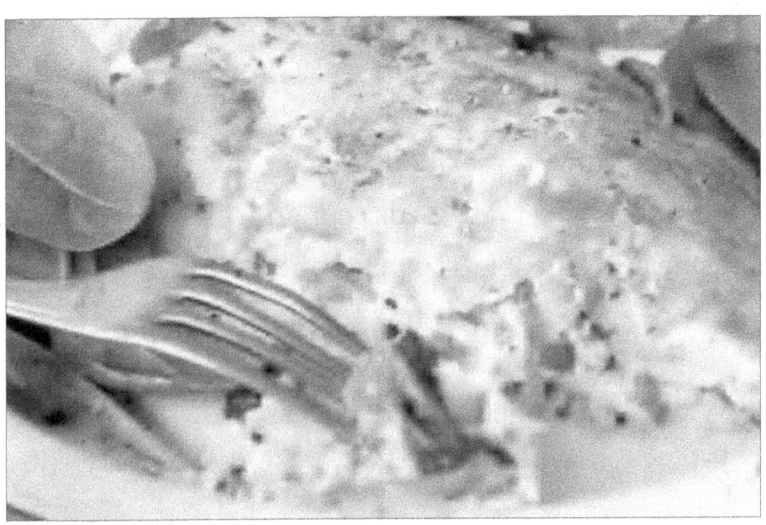

Servings: 2

### Ingredients

- 2 tbsp olive oil

- 5 oz cooked shrimp or seafood mix

- red chili pepper

- garlic cloves (optional)

- ½ tsp fennel seeds or ground cumin

- ½ cup mayonnaise

- 1 tbsp fresh or dried chives

- 6 eggs

- 2 tbsp olive oil or butter Salt and pepper to taste

## Directions:

1. Preheat broiler.

2. Broil shrimp or seafood mix in olive oil with minced garlic, chili, fennel seeds, cumin, salt, and pepper. Set aside and let cool to room temperature.

3. Add mayo and chives to the cooled mixture.

4. Whisk eggs together and season with salt and pepper. Fry in a non-stick skillet with plenty of butter or oil.

5. Add seafood mixture when the omelet is almost ready, then fold.

6. Lower heat and allow to set completely. Serve immediately.

## Macros

- 83g fat

- 27g protein

- 4g carbs

- 872 calories

# LUNCH

## KETO ASIAN AGE STIR-FRY

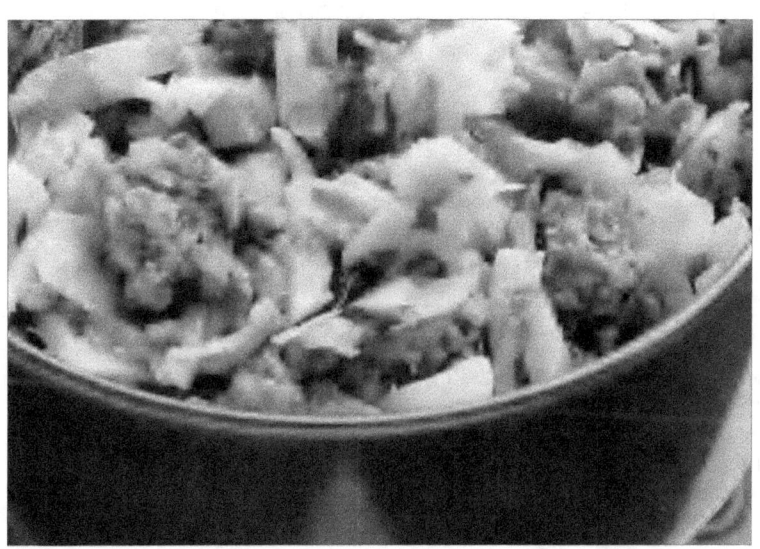

Servings : 4

### Ingredients

- 25 oz. green cabbage

- 5 oz. butter

- 20 oz. ground beef 1 tsp salt

- 1 tsp onion powder

- ¼ tsp ground black pepper

- tbsp white wine vinegar

- garlic cloves

- scallions, in slices

- 1 tsp chili flakes

- 1 tbsp fresh ginger, finely chopped or grated

- 1 tbsp sesame oil

- Wasabi mayonnaise

- 1 cup mayonnaise

- ½ - 1 tbsp wasabi paste

## Directions:

1. Shred the cabbage finely using a sharp knife or a food processor.

2. Fry the cabbage in 2–3 ounces (60–90 g) butter in a large frying or wok pan on mediumhigh heat, but don't let the cabbage turn brown. It takes a while for the cabbage to soften.

3. Add spices and vinegar. Stir and fry for a couple of minutes more. Put the cabbage in a bowl.

4. Melt the rest of the butter in the same frying pan. Add garlic, chili flakes, and ginger and sauté for a few minutes.

5. Add ground meat and brown until the meat is thoroughly cooked and most of the juices have evaporated. Lower the heat a little.

6. Add scallions and cabbage to the meat. Stir until everything is hot. Add salt and pepper to taste, and top with the sesame oil before serving.

7. Mix together the wasabi mayonnaise by starting with a small amount of wasabi and adding more until the flavor is just right. Serve the stir-fry warm with a dollop of wasabi mayonnaise on top.

## Macros

- 93g fat

- 33g protein

- 10g carbs

# DINNER

## KETO CHICKEN WITH HERB

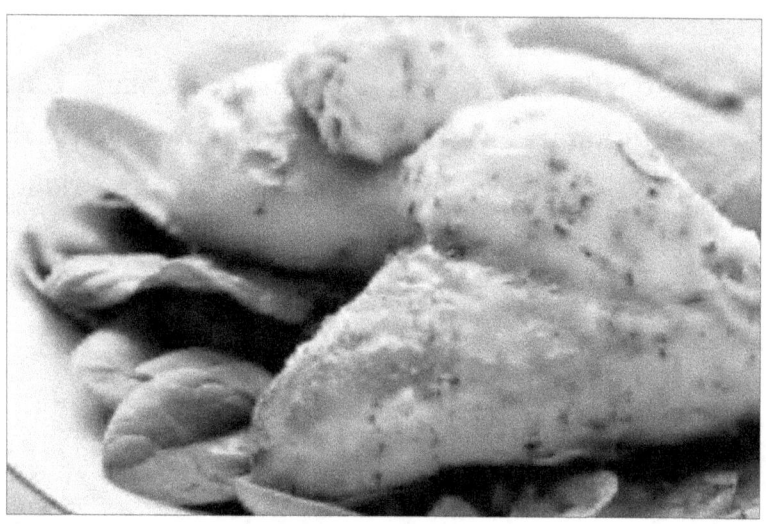

Servings: 4

## <u>Ingredients</u>

- Fried chicken

- 4 chicken breasts 1/6 oz. butter or olive oil salt and pepper

- Herb butter

- 51/3 oz. butter, at room temperature

- 1 garlic clove

- ½ tsp garlic powder

- 4 tbsp chopped fresh parsley

- 1 tsp lemon juice

- ½ tsp salt

- Leafy greens

- 8 oz. leafy greens, for example, baby spinach

## Directions:

1. Take the butter out of the fridge and bring to room temperature.

2. Start with the herb butter. Mix all ingredients thoroughly in a small bowl and let sit until it's time to serve.

3. Season the chicken with salt and pepper. Fry in butter or oil on medium heat until the fillets are cooked through, and register 165°F (75°C) with a meat thermometer. Lower the temperature towards the end to avoid dry chicken fillets.

4. Serve the chicken on a bed of leafy greens and place a generous amount of herb butter on top.

## Macros

- 64g fat

- 63g protein

- 2g carbs

- 841 calories

# THURSDAY
# BREAKFAST

## KETOQUE MONSIEUR

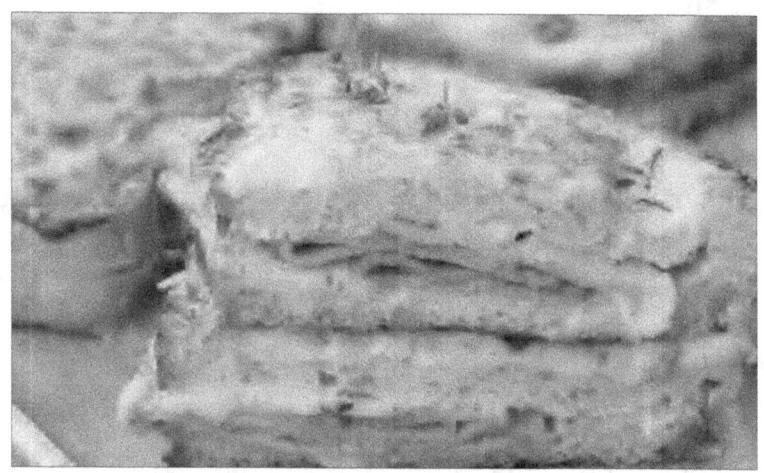

Servings: 4

## Ingredients

- 8 oz cottage cheese

- 4 eggs

- 1 tbsp ground psyllium husk powder

- tbsp butter or coconut oil for frying

- 1/3 oz smoked deli ham

- 5 1/3 oz cheddar cheese

- ½ finely chopped red onion (optional)

- ½ oz lettuce

- tbsp olive oil

- ½ tbsp red wine vinegar Salt and pepper

## Directions:

1. Whisk the eggs together in a bowl, then mix in the cottage cheese. Add ground psyllium husk powder while stirring to incorporate it smoothly, without lumps. Let the mixture rest for five minutes until the batter is set.

2. Place the frying pan over medium heat. Add a generous amount of butter and fry batter like small pancakes for about 2 minutes on each side, until they are golden. Make two pancakes per serving. 3. Assemble a sandwich with sliced ham and cheese between two of the warm pancakes. Add finely chopped onion on top.

3. Wash and tear the lettuce. Mix oil, vinegar, salt and pepper into a simple vinaigrette.

4. Serve the Croque Monsieur warm beside lettuce dressed with the vinaigrette.

## Macros

- 92g fat

- 54g protein

- 8g carbs

- 1082 calories

# LUNCH

## KETO ITALIAN CABBAGE STIR

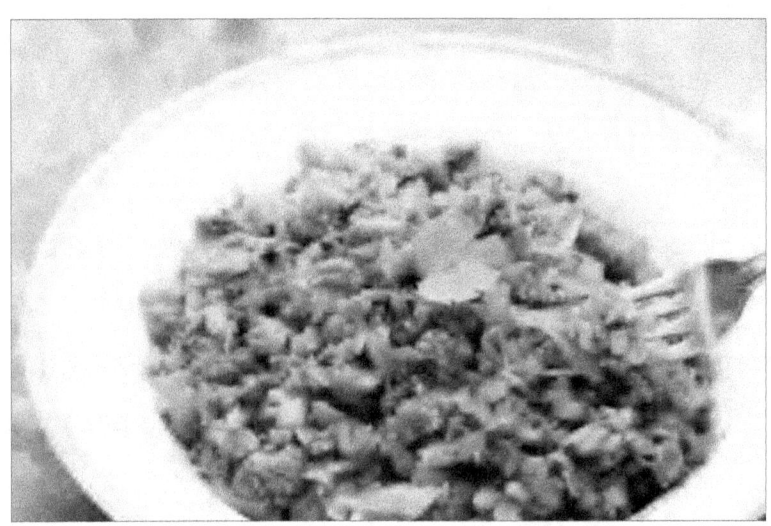

Servings: 4

### Ingredients

- 25 oz. green cabbage

- 51/3 oz. butter

- 20 oz. ground beef

- 1 tsp salt

- 1 tsp onion powder

- ¼ tsp pepper

- tbsp white wine vinegar 1 tbsp tomato paste

- garlic cloves, finely chopped

- oz. leeks, thinly sliced

- ½ cup fresh basil

- 1 cup mayonnaise or sour cream, for serving

## Directions:

1. Shred the green cabbage finely with a cheese slicer, sharp knife or in a food processor.

2. Fry the cabbage in about half of the butter (or substitute olive oil) in a large frying pan or wok on medium heat for about 10 minutes, or until just softened.

3. Add vinegar, salt, onion powder, and pepper. Stir and fry for 2-3 minutes, or until well incorporated. Reserve sautéed cabbage to a bowl.

4. Heat the rest of the butter or oil in the pan. Add the garlic and leeks, and sauté for a minute.

5. Add meat, and continue frying until cooked through. Sauté until most of the liquid has evaporated.

6. Add tomato paste and mix well. Lower the heat a little and add reserved cabbage and fresh basil. Stir until cooked through.

7. Adjust seasoning and serve with a dollop of sour cream or mayonnaise and perhaps even a green salad.

## Macros

- 91g fat
- 33g protein
- 9g carbs
- 1003 calories

# DINNER

## KETO SALMON WITH PESTO

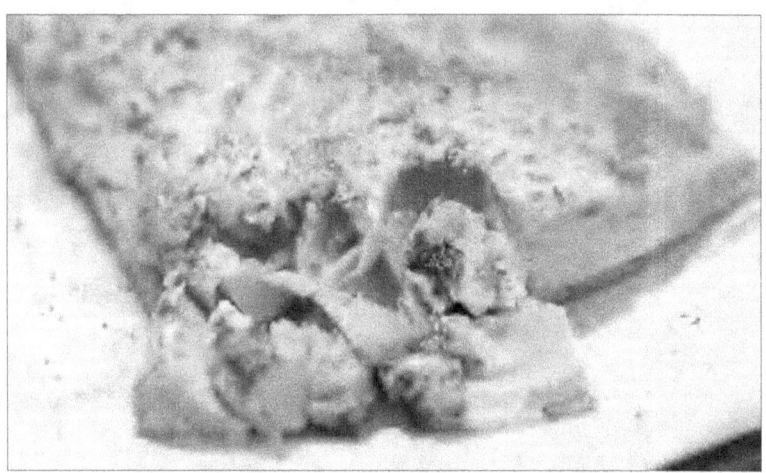

Servings: 4

### <u>Ingredients</u>

- 25 oz. salmon

- 1 cup mayonnaise or sour cream

- tbsp green pesto or red pesto

- oz. grated parmesan cheese

- 1 lb fresh spinach 1/6 oz. butter or olive oil salt and pepper

## Directions:

1. Preheat the oven to 400°F (200°C).

2. Grease a baking dish with half of the butter or oil. Salt and pepper the salmon fillets and place them in the prepared baking dish, skin-side down.

3. Mix mayonnaise, pesto, and parmesan cheese and spread over the salmon.

4. Bake for 15–20 minutes, or until the salmon is done and flakes easily with a fork.

5. Meanwhile, sauté the spinach in remaining butter or oil until it's wilted, about 2 minutes.

6. Season with salt and pepper.

7. Serve immediately with the oven-baked salmon.

## Macros

- 78g fat
- 45g protein
- 3g carbs
- 902 calories

# FRIDAY

# BREAKFAST

## KETO OVEN PANCAKE WITH BACON AND ONION RECIPE

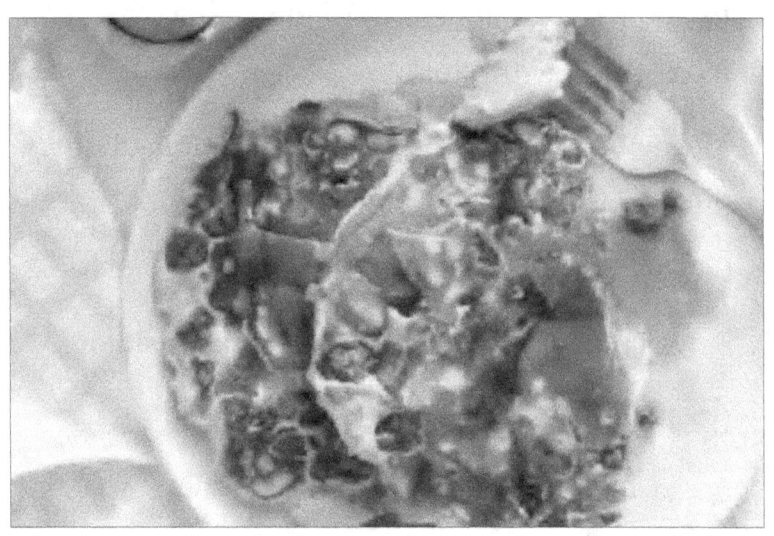

Servings:4

### Ingredients

- 3 ½ oz turkey

- ½ yellow onion

- 2 tbsp butter to fry in

- 4 eggs

- 1 cup heavy whipping cream

- ½ cup cottage cheese

- ½ cup almond flour

- 1 tbsp ground psyllium husk powder

- 1 tsp baking powder

- 1 tsp salt

- 1 tbsp chopped parsley for garnish (optional)

## Directions:

1. Preheat the oven to 350°F (175°C).

2. Slice the bacon and onion. Heat butter in a frying pan and add bacon and onion. Fry until the onion is soft and the bacon starts getting crispy.

3. In a bowl, whisk together eggs, cottage cheese, and cream. Add almond flour, psyllium husk, baking powder, and salt. Whisk until thoroughly combined. Let it rest for a couple of minutes.

4. Pour the pancake batter into a greased baking pan and sprinkle the fried bacon and onions on top.

5. Bake for 20-25 minutes. It's ready when it's puffy, golden brown and the center has set.

## <u>Macros</u>

- 50g fat
- 16g protein
- 5g carbs
- 545 calories

# LUNCH

## KETO CHOPS WITH GREEN BEANS AND AVOCADO RECIPE

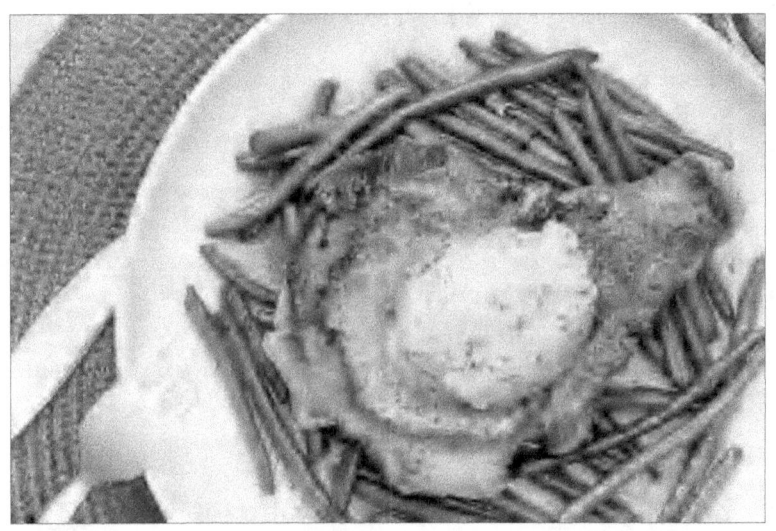

Servings: 4

### Ingredients

- Pork shoulder chops

- 2 tbsp mild chipotle paste

- 2 tbsp olive oil

- ½ tsp salt

- 4 pork shoulder chops

- Garlic butter

- 4¼ oz. butter, at room temperature

- garlic clove

- ½ tsp salt

- ¼ tsp ground black pepper

- ¼ tsp paprika powder

- Green beans and avocado

- tbsp olive oil

- 10 oz. fresh green beans

- ½ tsp salt

- ¼ tsp ground black pepper

- 2 avocados 6 scallions fresh cilantro (optional) pepper to taste

## Directions:

1. Mix chipotle paste, oil, and salt in a small bowl.

2. Brush the meat with the marinade and let sit for 15 minutes. You can also marinate the meat in a plastic bag for 30 minutes or more in the fridge.

3. Preheat the oven to 400°F (200°C). Grill the marinated meat on a rack on a baking sheet in the oven for 20–30

minutes until the meat is thoroughly done. Turn after 10-15 minutes.

4. Meanwhile, prepare the garlic butter and the beans. Press the garlic clove, mix with butter and spices and set aside.

5. Heat the oil in a frying pan. Sauté the beans for about 5 minutes on medium high heat until they have turned a nice color. Lower the heat towards the end, and add spices.

6. Chop the onion finely. Peel and remove the pit from the avocado and mash the flesh coarsely with a fork. Stir onion and avocado into the beans. Season with salt and pepper to taste. Top with a handful of finely chopped cilantro.

## Macros

- 78g fat
- 39g protein
- 6g carbs
- 901 calories

# DINNER

## KETO BAKED SALMON WITH LEMON AND BUTTER RECIPE

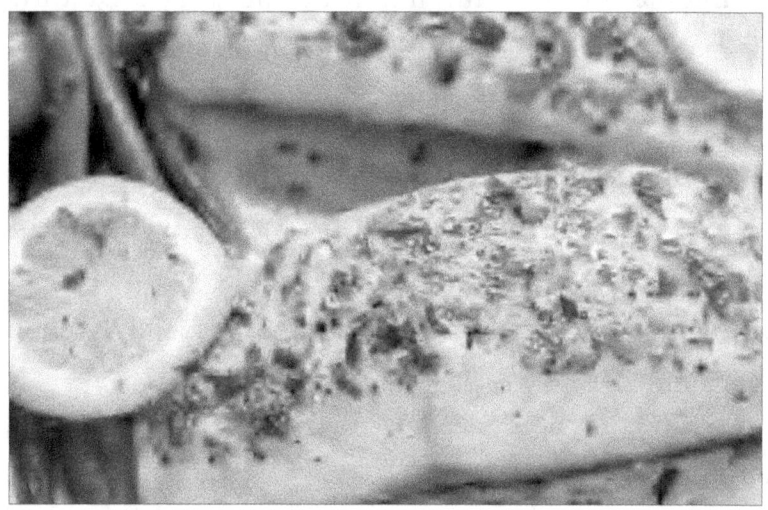

Servings: 6

### Ingredients

- tbsp olive oil

- lbs salmon 1 tsp sea salt ground black pepper

- 7 oz. butter

- 1 lemon

## Directions:

1. Preheat the oven to 400°F (200°C).

2. Grease a large baking dish with olive oil. Place the salmon, with the skin-side down, in the prepared baking dish. Generously season with salt and pepper.

3. Slice the lemon thinly and place on top of the salmon. Cover with half of the butter in thin slices.

4. Bake on the middle rack for about 20–30 minutes, or until the salmon is opaque and flakes easily with a fork.

5. 5. Heat the rest of the butter in a small saucepan until it starts to bubble. Remove from heat and let cool a little. Gently add some lemon juice.

6. 6. Serve the fish with the lemon butter and a side dish of your choice.

## Macros

- 49g fat
- 31g protein
- 1g carbs
- 573 calories

# SATURDAY BREAKFAST

## KETO OVER PANCAKE WITH BACON AND ONION RECIPE

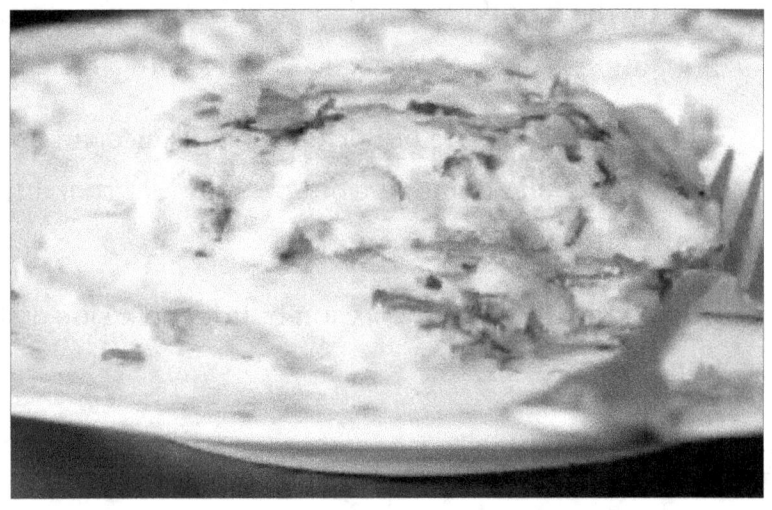

Servings: 4

## Ingredients

- 3 ½ oz turkey or pork bacon

- eggs

- tomatoes

- 1 tsp salt black pepper

- 3 oz. butter or olive oil

## Directions:

1 . Crack the eggs into a mixing bowl, add salt and black pepper to your liking. Whisk well with a fork until fully combined. Add basil and stir.

2 . Cut the tomatoes into halves or slices, then fry them for a few minutes.

3 . 3. Pour the egg batter on top of the tomatoes. Wait until batter is slightly set before adding the mozzarella cheese.

4 . 4. Lower the heat and let the omelet set, then serve immediately.

## Macros

- 50g fat

- 16g protein

- 5g carbs

- 545 calories

# LUNCH

## KETO FISH CASSEROLE WITH MUSHROOMS AND FRENCH MUSTARD RECIPE

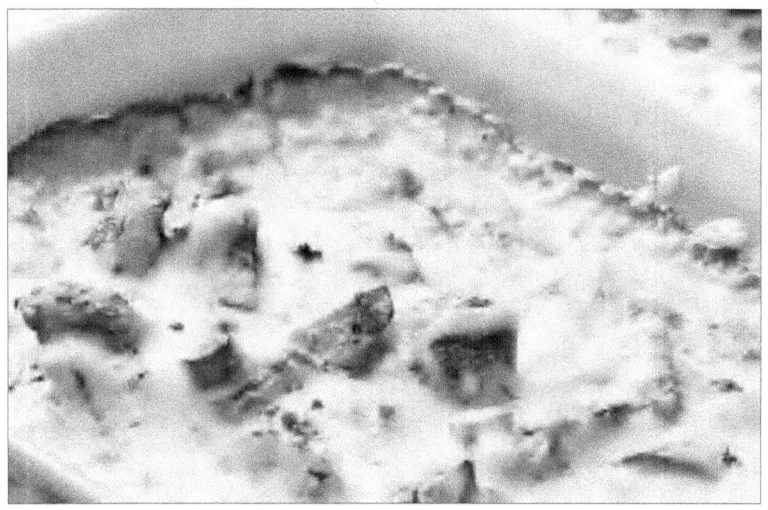

Servings: 6

### Ingredients

- 15 oz. mushrooms

- 3 oz. butter 1 tsp salt pepper, to taste 2 tbsp fresh parsley

- 2 cups heavy whipping cream

- 2 tbsp Dijon mustard

- 8 oz. shredded cheese

- 25 oz. white fish, for example, cod

- 20 oz. broccoli or cauliflower

- 3 oz. butter or olive oil

## Directions:

1. Preheat the oven to 350°F (175°C).

2. Cut the mushrooms into wedges. Fry in butter until the mushrooms have softened, about 5 minutes. Add salt, pepper, and parsley.

3. Pour in the heavy cream and mustard and lower the heat. Let simmer for 5-10 minutes to reduce the sauce a bit.

4. Season the fish with salt and pepper and place in a greased baking dish. Sprinkle 3/4 of the cheese on and pour the creamed mushrooms on top. Top with the remaining cheese.

5. Bake for about 30 minutes if the fish is frozen, or slightly less if it's fresh. Probe with a sharp knife after 20 minutes; the fish is done if it flakes easily with a fork. And remember that the fish will continue to cook even after you have taken it out of the oven.

6. Meanwhile, make the side dish. Cut the broccoli or cauliflower into florets. Boil in lightly salted water for a few minutes. Strain off the water and add olive oil or butter. Mash coarsely with a wooden spoon or fork.

7. Season with salt and pepper and serve with the fish.

## Macros

- 71g fat
- 39g protein
- 9g carbs
- 828 calories

# DINNER

## KETO SALMON TANDOORI WITH CUCUMBER SAUCE RECIPE

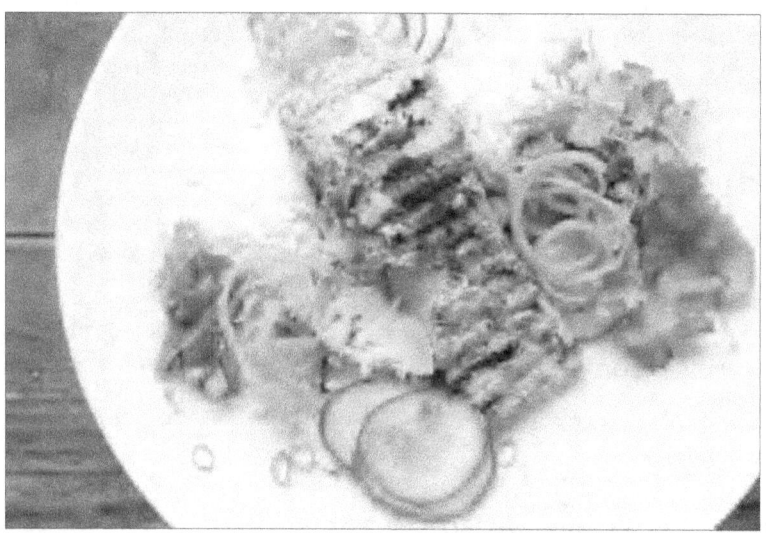

Servings: 4

### Ingredients

- 20 oz. salmon, in pieces

- 2 tbsp tandoori seasoning

- 2 tbsp olive oil or coconut oil

- Cucumber sauce

- ¾ cup mayonnaise or sour cream

- ½ cucumber, shredded

- 2 garlic cloves, minced

- ½ lime, the juice

- ½ tsp salt (optional)

- Crispy salad

- 5 oz. arugula lettuce

- 1 yellow bell pepper

- 3 scallions

- 2 avocados

- Juice from 1 lime

## Directions:

1. Heat the oven to 350°F (175°C).

2. Mix tandoori seasoning with oil and cover the salmon.

3. Place in the oven for 15–20 minutes, or until the salmon flakes easily with a fork.

4. Mix crushed garlic, lime juice, shredded cucumber (squeeze out the water first) and mayonnaise and/or sour cream in a bowl.

5. Chop bell peppers, scallions, and avocados. Combine with the arugula on a platter.

6. Drizzle with lime juice.

7. Serve salmon on the salad, and top with cucumber sauce.

## <u>Macros</u>

- 73g fat
- 35g protein
- 8g carbs
- 847 calories

# SUNDAY BREAKFAST

## KETO EGGS ON THE

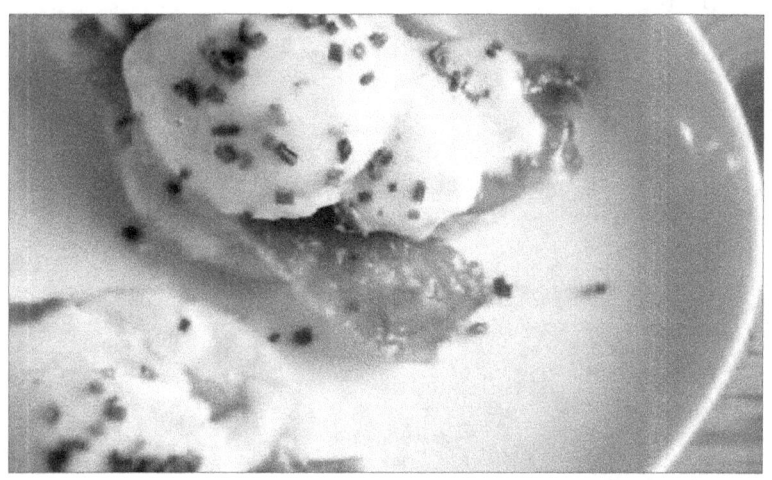

Servings:6

## Ingredients

- 12 eggs

- Salt and pepper to taste

- 4 oz cooked bacon

## Directions:

1. Preheat oven to 400°F.

2. Place cupcake liners in a muffin tin to avoid the eggs sticking to the tin.

3. Crack one egg in each liner and add crumbled bacon or substitute another filling.

4. Season to taste.

5. Bake for about 15 minutes or until eggs is cooked.

## Macros

- 16g fat
- 13g protein
- 1g carbs
- 205 calories

# LUNCH

## KETO INDIAN CABBAGE STIR

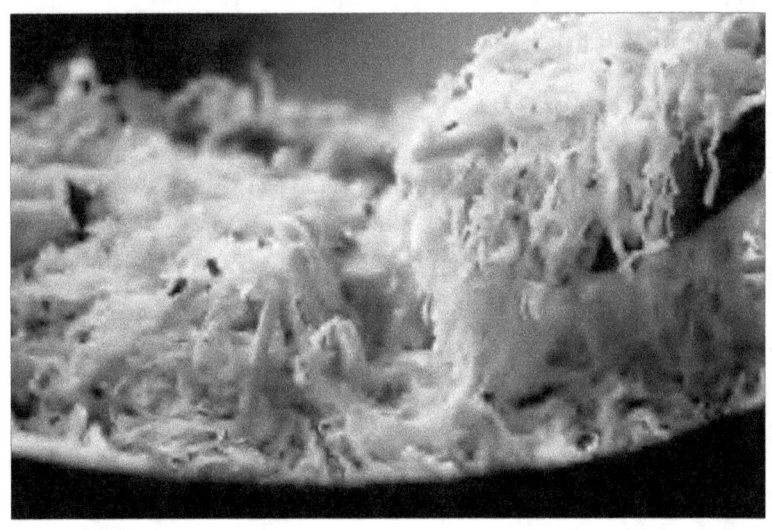

Servings:

### <u>Ingredients</u>

- 25 oz. green cabbage

- 51/3 oz. butter

- 20 oz. ground pork or ground lamb

- tsp salt

- garlic cloves

- 1 tsp onion powder

- ¼ tsp ground black pepper

- 1 tbsp white wine vinegar

- 1 tbsp red curry paste

- ½ yellow onion, finely chopped

- ½ cup fresh cilantro

- 1 cup mayonnaise

## Directions:

- Shred the cabbage with a knife or in a food processor as finely as possible.

- Fry the cabbage in half of the butter in a large frying pan or wok on medium-high heat until softened, about 5-6 minutes.

- Add spices and vinegar. Sauté until fragrant. Place the cabbage in a bowl, and reserve.

- Melt the rest of the butter in the same pan. Add garlic, onion, and curry paste. Sauté for 1 minute. Add ground meat and sauté until the meat is cooked through and most of the liquid has evaporated.

- Lower the heat a little and add the cabbage back to the pan. Stir until everything is warmed through.

- Finish seasoning with salt and pepper to taste. Garnish with fresh cilantro before serving with a dollop of mayonnaise or sour cream.

## Macros

- 97g fat

- 31g protein

- 10g carbs

- 1040 calories

# DINNER

## SLOW-COOKED KETO PORK ROAST WITH CREAMY GRAVY RECIPE

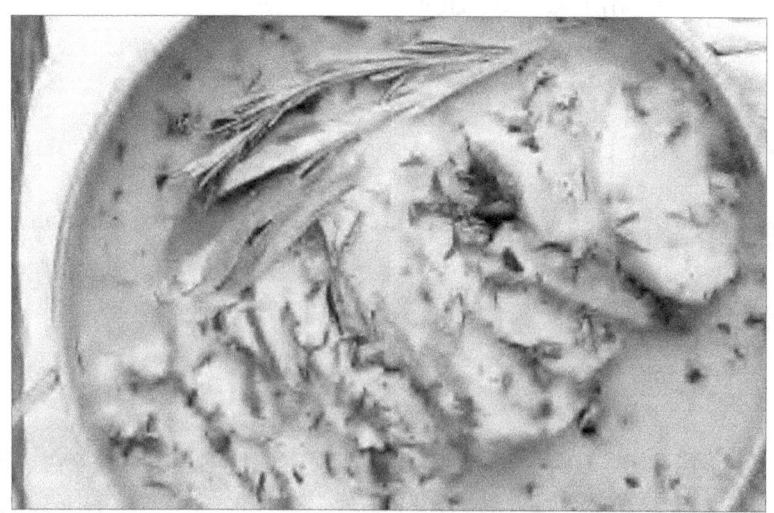

Servings:6

### <u>Ingredients</u>

- 30 oz. pork shoulder or pork roast

- ½ tbsp salt

- 1 bay leaf

- 5 black peppercorns

- 2½ cups water

- 2 tsp dried thyme or dried rosemary

- 2 garlic cloves

- 1½ oz. fresh ginger

- 1 tbsp olive oil or coconut oil

- 1 tbsp paprika powder

- ½ tsp ground black pepper

- Creamy gravy

- 1½ cups heavy whipping cream juices from the roast

## Directions:

1. Preheat the oven to low heat at 200°F (100°C).

2. Place the meat in a deep baking dish and season with salt. Add water to cover 1/3 of the meat. Add bay leaf, peppercorns, and thyme. Place the baking dish in the oven for 7–8 hours, covered with aluminum foil.

3. If you're using a slow cooker, do the same thing in step 2 but only add 1 cup of water. Cook for 8 hours on low or 4 hours on high.

4. Remove the meat from the baking dish, and reserve the pan juices in a separate pan.

5. Turn the oven up to 450°F (220°C).

6. Grate or finely chop garlic and ginger in a small bowl. Add oil, herbs, and pepper and stir well to combine.

7. Rub the meat with the garlic/herb mixture.

8. Return the meat to the baking dish, and roast for about 10–15 minutes, or until golden brown.

9. Cut the meat into thin slices and serve with the creamy gravy and side dishes of your choice.

## Macros

- 51g fat

- 28g protein □ 3g carbs

- 586 calories

# CONCLUSION

For many people, a ketogenic diet is a great option for weight loss. It is very different and allows the person on the diet to eat a diet that consists of foods that you may not expect.

So the ketogenic diet, or keto, is a diet that consists of very low carbs and high fat. How many diets are there where you can start your day off with bacon and eggs, loads of it, then follow it up with chicken wings for lunch and then steak and broccoli for dinner. That may sound too good to be true for many. Well on this diet this is a great day of eating and you followed the rules perfectly with that meal plan.

When you eat a very low amount of carbs your body gets put into a state of ketosis. What this means is your body burns fat for energy. How low of a number of carbs do you need to eat in order to get into ketosis? Well, it varies from person to person, but it is a safe bet to stay under 25 net carbs. Many would suggest that when you are in the "induction phase" which is when you are actually putting your body into ketosis, you should stay under 10 net carbs.

If you aren't sure what net carbs are, let me help you. Net carbs are the number of carbs you eat minus the amount of dietary fiber. So if on the day you eat a total of 35 grams of net carbs and 13 grams of dietary fiber, your net carbs for the day would be 22. Simple enough, right?

So besides weight loss what else is good about keto? Well, many people talk about their improved mental clarity on when on the diet. Another benefit is having an increase in energy. Yet another is a decreased appetite.

One thing to worry about when going on the ketogenic diet is something called "keto flu." Not everyone experiences this, but for this that do, it can be tough. You will feel lethargic and you may have a headache. It won't last very long. When you feel this way make sure you get plenty of water and rest to get through it.

If this sounds like the kind of diet you would be interested in, then what are you waiting for?

Dive head first into keto. You won't believe the results you get in such a short amount of time.

www.ingramcontent.com/pod-product-compliance
Lightning Source LLC
Chambersburg PA
CBHW070416290526
45791CB00005B/1721